HEMOGLOBIN:
STRUCTURE, FUNCTION, EVOLUTION, AND PATHOLOGY

The Benjamin/Cummings Series in the Life Sciences

F. J. Ayala
POPULATION AND EVOLUTIONARY GENETICS: A PRIMER (1982)

F. J. Ayala and J. A. Kiger, Jr.
MODERN GENETICS (1980)

F. J. Ayala and J. W. Valentine
EVOLVING: THE THEORY AND PROCESSES OF ORGANIC EVOLUTION (1979)

M. G. Barbour, J. H. Burk, and W. D. Pitts
TERRESTRIAL PLANT ECOLOGY (1980)

L. L. Cavalli-Sforza
ELEMENTS OF HUMAN GENETICS, second edition (1977)

R. E. Dickerson and I. Geis
THE STRUCTURE AND ACTION OF PROTEINS (1969)

R. E. Dickerson and I. Geis
HEMOGLOBIN (1983)

P. B. Hackett, J. A. Fuchs, and J. Messing
RECOMBINANT DNA TECHNIQUES

L. E. Hood, I. L. Weissman, W. B. Wood, and J. H. Wilson
IMMUNOLOGY, second edition (1983)

L. E. Hood, J. H. Wilson, and W. B. Wood
MOLECULAR BIOLOGY OF EUCARYOTIC CELLS (1975)

A. L. Lehninger
BIOENERGETICS: THE MOLECULAR BASIS OF BIOLOGICAL ENERGY TRANSFORMATIONS, second edition (1971)

S. E. Luria, S. J. Gould, and S. Singer
A VIEW OF LIFE (1981)

A. P. Spence
BASIC HUMAN ANATOMY (1982)

A. P. Spence and E.B. Mason
HUMAN ANATOMY AND PHYSIOLOGY, second edition (1983)

G. J. Tortora, B. R. Funke, and C. L. Case
MICROBIOLOGY: AN INTRODUCTION (1982)

J. D. Watson, J. A. Steitz, Nancy Hopkins, and J. W. Roberts
MOLECULAR BIOLOGY OF THE GENE, fourth edition (1984)

I. L. Weissman, L. E. Hood, and W. B. Wood
ESSENTIAL CONCEPTS IN IMMUNOLOGY (1978)

N. K. Wessells
TISSUE INTERACTIONS AND DEVELOPMENT (1977)

W. B. Wood, J. H. Wilson, R. M. Benbow, and L. E. Hood
BIOCHEMISTRY: A PROBLEMS APPROACH, second edition (1981)

HEMOGLOBIN:
STRUCTURE, FUNCTION, EVOLUTION, AND PATHOLOGY

RICHARD E. DICKERSON
University of California at Los Angeles

IRVING GEIS
University of Chicago

THE BENJAMIN/CUMMINGS PUBLISHING COMPANY, INC.
MENLO PARK, CALIFORNIA • READING, MASSACHUSETTS
LONDON • AMSTERDAM • DON MILLS, ONTARIO • SYDNEY

Sponsoring Editor: Philip Hagopian
Production Manager: Margaret Moore
Senior Production Coordinator: Karen Bierstedt
Interior Design: Paul Quin

Copyright © 1983 by The Benjamin/Cummings Publishing Company, Inc.
Illustrations copyright © Irving Geis with the following exceptions: Figures 2.1, 2.11, 3.8, 3.12, 3.13, 3.14, 3.15, 3.17, 4.1, 4.5, 4.8, 4.9, 4.10, 4.11, 4.13, 4.28, 4.29, 4.30, 4.31b (top).

Information regarding permission to reproduce the illustrations may be obtained from the copyright holder: Irving Geis, 4700 Broadway, New York, NY 10040.

Library of Congress Cataloging in Publication Data

Dickerson, Richard Earl.
   Hemoglobin : structure, function, evolution, and
pathology.

   (The Benjamin/Cummings series in the life sciences)
   Includes bibliographies and index.
   1. Hemoglobin.   2. Hemoglobinopathy.   I. Geis,
Irving.   II. Title.   III. Series.   [DNLM: 1. Hemoglobins.
WH 190 D549h]
QP96 5.D53   1983   612'.1111   82-17741
ISBN 0-8053-2411-9

abcdefghij–HA–898765432

The Benjamin/Cummings Publishing Company, Inc.
2727 Sand Hill Road
Menlo Park, California 94025

ABOUT THE AUTHORS

Richard E. Dickerson is Professor of Biochemistry and Geophysics at the University of California at Los Angeles. Born in Illinois in 1931, he earned a B.S. in chemistry from the Carnegie Institute of Technology (now Carnegie-Mellon University) in Pittsburgh in 1953 and a Ph.D. in physical chemistry in 1957 from the University of Minnesota, where he worked with William N. Lipscomb on crystal structure analysis of boron hydrides.

After a year's postdoctoral stay at Leeds University in England, he moved south to Cambridge University to join John Kendrew and Max Perutz in their projects to solve the first x-ray analyses of crystalline proteins—myoglobin and hemoglobin. Dickerson and another postdoctoral fellow, Bror Strandberg, solved the structure of sperm whale myoglobin at 2 Å resolution, enabling the complete protein chain to be traced for the first time.

After four years as Assistant Professor in Chemistry at the University of Illinois, Dickerson moved to Caltech as Associate Professor in 1963, and became Professor of Physical Chemistry in 1968. At Caltech his main areas of research were in structural analysis and comparative evolution of vertebrate and bacterial cytochromes c but also included analysis of the enzyme trypsin and the foundations of his current activity in DNA structure analysis.

In 1981 he and his team moved to UCLA, where their main research emphasis in the Molecular Biology Institute is on structure analyses of short oligomers of DNA and their complexes with antitumor drugs and DNA-binding proteins such as repressors. As a member of the UCLA Institute of Geophysics and Planetary Physics, he maintains an interest in chemical and molecular evolution and the origin of life. He and his wife are just sending the last of five children through college. His principal nonscientific interests are ancient and nineteenth-century history and Baroque and Russian opera.

Irving Geis began his career as a scientific illustrator in New York City in 1938 with drawings for *Fortune* magazine. Since 1948 he has contributed illustrations to *Scientific American*, notably paintings and drawings of protein molecules worked out in collaboration with the authors: myoglobin with John Kendrew in 1961, lysozyme with David Phillips in 1966, and cytochrome c with Richard Dickerson in 1972.

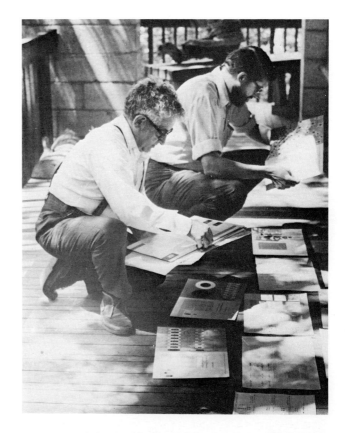

Hemoglobin is the third Dickerson/Geis collaboration for Benjamin/Cummings. The other two, in order of appearance, are *The Structure and Action of Proteins* (1969) and *Chemistry, Matter, and the Universe* (1976).

Geis was a student of architecture at the Georgia Institute of Technology and the University of Pennsylvania, where he received a Fine Arts degree in 1929. His present major interest is depicting macromolecular structures, reprints of which appear in major biology and biochemistry textbooks. He is an Associate in the Department of Biophysics and Theoretical Biology at the University of Chicago, where he acts as consultant on the molecular basis of sickle hemoglobin assembly.

On the lighter side, Geis is a cartoonist and collector of classic comic art (Paris in the 1890s and New York in the 1920s). He is the illustrator and co-author, with Darrell Huff, of the amusing bestseller *How to Lie with Statistics,* now in its 34th printing.

To Max F. Perutz, who laid the foundation for an entire field.

When the early explorers of America made their first landfall, they had the unforgettable experience of glimpsing a New World that no European had ever seen before. Moments such as this—first visions of new worlds—are one of the main attractions of exploration. From time to time scientists are privileged to share excitements of the same kind. Such a moment arrived for my colleagues and me one Sunday morning in 1957, when we looked at something no one before us had seen: a three-dimensional picture of a protein molecule in all its complexity.

John C. Kendrew, 1961

PREFACE

There are three good reasons for writing a book about hemoglobin. To begin with, it and its cousin myoglobin were *first*—the very first proteins for which three-dimensional structures were worked out by x-ray methods, and nearly the first in amino acid sequence determination also. In a world that values explorers and pioneers, the first of any new field invariably has a special interest. Moreover, hemoglobin has the advantage of familiarity. People for whom alpha-ketoglutarate dehydrogenase has no charms immediately recognize hemoglobin as the essential constituent of blood, without which human life would be impossible. Most important of all, perhaps, is the fact that with this one family of macromolecules—hemoglobin and myoglobin—one can illustrate nearly every important feature of protein structure, function, and evolution: principles of amino acid sequence and protein folding, a mechanism of activity that resembles that found in enzymes although not itself catalytic, specificity in the recognition and binding of large and small molecules, subunit motion and allosteric control in regulating activity, gene structure and genetic control, and the effects of point mutations on molecular behavior. Finally, the widespread occurrence of globins and the vast body of amino acid sequence information that has been built up from many species makes the globins the system of choice in a beginning study of molecular evolution, a position only challenged by the electron transport protein cytochrome *c*.

This book has two related but distinct roots: a planned revision of our "Structure and Action of Proteins," first published in 1969, and a course in molecular evolution developed first at Caltech but given over the past four years at the University of Southern California and UCLA as well. When we wrote the first edition of "Proteins" in 1968, three-dimensional structures were known for only eight proteins. Ten years later when the revision process began, this number had risen to more than 150! Obviously what was called for in the second edition was not an exposition of 150 different structures, but a critical analysis of families of evolutionarily related proteins. The globin family was an obvious paradigm for other, less well-studied families. What had begun as an exposition of principles of protein folding, activity, and evolution, using the globin family as an example, grew by slow but unmistakable steps into a book on hemoglobin in its own right. The short book providing a comprehensive overview of protein structure and function remains to be written.

The present book on hemoglobin structure, function, evolution, and pathology also grew directly out of a one-term or one-semester course on molecular evolution, addressed to upper division undergraduates and beginning graduate students. This book contains the material of roughly the first 40 percent of the course, as it developed over several years of trial and error, in which fundamental principles were developed using the globin family as an example. These principles then were reiterated and extended with cytochrome *c* and other electron transport proteins, and the final third of the course featured a survey of other and less well-documented (to date) families of proteins: serine and acid proteases, dehydrogenases, and other enzymes of intermediary metabolism, immunoglobulins, and viruses, with a concluding look at attempts at functional classification of protein structures. *Hemoglobin* is essentially the core of this course in Molecular Evolution—it sets out the general principles that then can be applied to other protein families, for which the students can turn to the original scientific literature.

The material in this book, therefore, has been thoroughly class-tested at three different institutions over a period of five years. It also has been tested against the most severe and critical audience of all: the investigators who were responsible for carrying out the original research. Individual chapters were sent out to many scientists, and we studied the slashed and tattered remnants with a view toward improving the presentation. Our philosophy, stated at the outset, was that we would not take offense at any suggestions made by the primary research workers, provided that they would not take offense at our decisions to ignore some of their suggestions. The arrangement seems to have worked well.

Among the people who have read and criticized portions of our book, we would like to acknowledge, in roughly geographical order: Max Perutz and Joyce Baldwin at Cambridge University, Cyrus Chothia of London University, Tom Maniatis, John Edsall, Franklin Bunn, and Martin Karplus of Harvard, Robert Shulman of Yale, Stuart Edelstein and Richard Crepeau of Cornell and Esther Breslow of Cornell Medical Center, James Manning of Rockefeller University, Arthur Bank, Johnathan Greer, John Bertles, and Beatrice Magdoff Fairchild of Columbia, William Poillon of Howard University, Robert Bookchin of Albert Einstein College of Medicine, Thomas Wellems of the University of Pennsylvania, Gary Ackers, Warner Love, Eduardo Padlan, and Samuel Charache of Johns Hopkins University and School of Medicine, Alan Schechter, Constance Noguchi, William Eaton, and Richard Feldman of the National Institutes of Health, William Brown, Chien Ho, and Irina Russu of Carnegie-Mellon University, Margaret Dayhoff of the Georgetown University Medical Center, Frank Gurd of Indiana University, Robert Josephs of the University of Chicago, Walter Fitch of the University of Wisconsin, Arthur Arnone and Joseph Walder of the University of Iowa, and Tsunehiro Takano of Osaka University.

Thanks are also due to Dee Barr for several years of retyping manuscripts, and to Lyris Schiller for drafting assistance during the five-year process of preparing illustrations. Phil Hagopian and Margaret Moore of the Benjamin/Cummings Publishing Company were indispensable as Editor and Production Editor in getting through a long development process.

As was mentioned at the beginning of this Preface, we did not actually set out to write this book at all—it developed a life of its own. We hope that it will prove as stimulating to read as it has been to write, and that we now can turn to the original goal: the short, one-volume introduction to protein structure.

Richard E. Dickerson and Irving Geis

CONTENTS

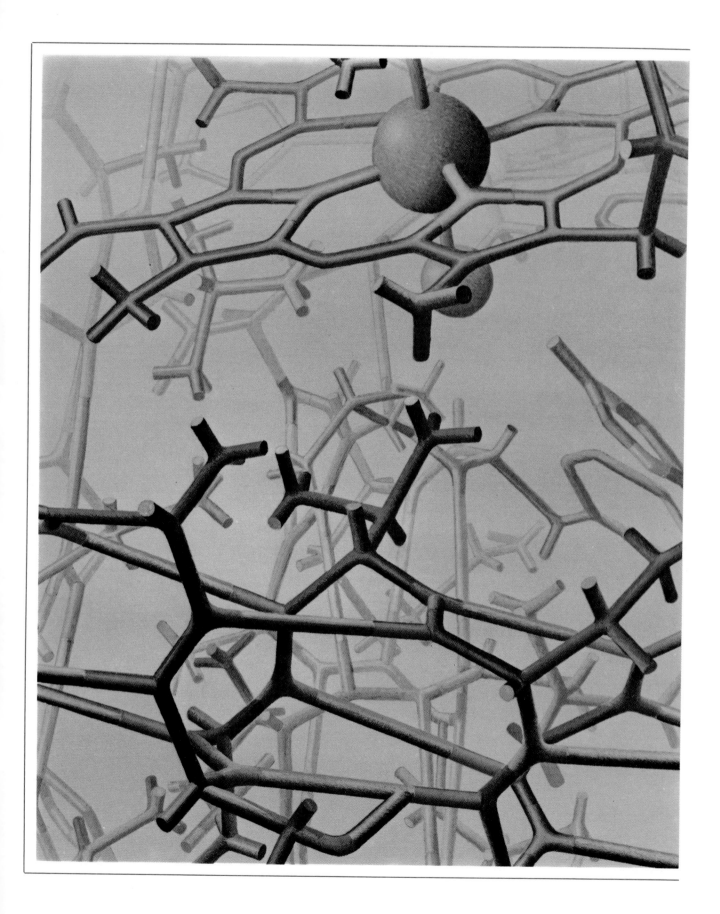

1 THE RULES OF THE GAME

← *The heme binding pocket in myoglobin. Understanding the molecular architecture of proteins began with the elucidation of myoglobin at the atomic level. The drawing at left shows a close-up view into the oxygen-binding heme pocket in the molecule of sperm whale myoglobin, a close relative of hemoglobin. In this "wire" model, chemical bonds are represented by sticks, and atoms are to be imagined at the intersections of the bonds. Only the central iron atom is shown explicitly, sitting in the middle of the flat heme group. A side chain from the protein attaches to the heme iron from the top, and the small sphere attached to it from below indicates where the oxygen molecule binds to myoglobin during storage in the tissues. For an overview of the entire molecule from Scientific American, see Figure 1.1.*

CHAPTER ONE

THE RULES
OF THE GAME

The American biochemist L. J. Henderson once described hemoglobin as "the second most interesting substance in the world" (1), a tantalizing comment in the same vein as the description of the Law as "the second oldest profession." Nevertheless, hemoglobin must surely be the most studied and discussed substance in the human body. Long before people were scientists in the modern sense, they were perceptive observers, and they noticed that an adequate quantity of blood was a prerequisite for survival. Blood was erroneously considered by some as the medium of heredity ("bloodlines") or of emotions ("sanguine humor" and "bad blood"). The Hippocratic school of medicine considered blood one of the four vital fluids, along with phlegm, black bile, and yellow bile, and thought that personality or temperament depended on the particular proportions of these four fluids or "humors." Aristotle taught that blood was manufactured from food in the liver and then pumped by the heart via the veins and capillaries to all parts of the body. Because the arteries emptied of blood after death, medieval anatomists thought that they were the separate carriers of vital airs or substances. (The term *artery,* probably derived from the Greek for "airway," was originally applied to the trachea as well.) "The vaynes bereth the nourysshyng blode, and the arteres the spyrytual blode" (R. Copland, *Guydon's Quest. Cyrurg.,* 1541). Not until the work of the English physician William Harvey (1578–1657) did people realize that both veins and arteries were part of a common mechanism for continuous circulation of blood.

But why was it so important that blood should circulate, and what was responsible for the red color of arterial blood and the purple color of blood from the veins? Ideas about the importance of oxygen for life, and the production of animal heat by controlled combustion or respiration, developed slowly in the eighteenth and nineteenth centuries. Not until 1864 was it shown by the English mathematician and physicist George Stokes that hemoglobin, the pigment of the blood, reversibly binds and and releases oxygen, changing color as it does so. Only then was the principal (but not the sole) physiological function of hemoglobin and of blood circulation appreciated. In 1904, Christian Bohr (the father of Niels Bohr) and his younger colleagues discovered that the amount of oxygen that hemoglobin was able to deliver to metabolizing tissues was linked to concentrations of carbon dioxide. This connection between oxygen binding and ultimately the protons derived from CO_2 is known today as the Bohr effect.

Hemoglobin has played an important role in the history of protein research. It is a relatively tough molecule, not easily destroyed by handling. More important, it is easy to obtain in large quantities without doing permanent damage to the donor. It was the first protein to be crystallized, by K. B. Reichert in 1849, and the first protein whose physiological purpose was known. A brave if premature essay in molecular evolution was made with hemoglobin in 1909 by E. T. Reichert and A. P. Brown, who attempted to use a comparison of hemoglobin crystal forms as a means of deducing phylogenetic relationships between species (2). Their approach was sound; only their data were inadequate. Had they had access to the amino acid sequence comparisons detailed in Chapter 3, then all the progress in molecular evolution described in Chapter 3 probably would have occurred a half-century earlier.

Hemoglobin was one of the first proteins to be purified to the point where its molecular weight and amino acid composition could be established accurately. This was crucial in leading, in the 1930s, to the demise of the old idea of protein as a colloidal mixture of polymers of no defined molecular weight or composition. A new concept arose, in which *a protein* was viewed as a definite compound, each molecule of which had exactly the same molecular weight and was built from the same amino acid subunits connected in the same order along a chain.

The means of deciphering the order of amino acids along a protein (or polypeptide) chain were not developed until 1951, when Fred Sanger obtained the amino acid sequence of insulin. The sequences for α and β chains of hemoglobin and its close relative myoglobin followed in the next few years. But in 1959–1960 there were even more dramatic developments: the first three-dimensional structure analyses of any proteins, those of myoglobin and hemoglobin, by x-ray diffraction methods. For the first time the molecular architecture of a protein was known, making it possible to build a detailed model in which every atom was located (Figure 1.1).

A close-up view of the oxygen-binding region of the myoglobin molecule is shown at the beginning of this chapter. We will have more to say about this molecule and hemoglobin all through this book. For the moment, let it be said only that the purpose of both proteins is to store and carry oxygen molecules, that the O_2 molecules bind to an iron atom situated at the heart of the molecule, and that the oxygen-binding properties of the iron atom are fine-tuned by surrounding it first with a flat ring to make a heme group, and then with a cage of folded protein chain. Perhaps the central question that this book will try to answer is this: What desirable effects does the protein chain have on the behavior of the iron atom, and how are these effects brought about?

Chapter 2 outlines the structures of myoglobin and hemoglobin in their oxygenated and deoxygenated states, and attempts to show how structure can account for the biochemical and physiological properties of the proteins. Chapter 3 discusses how myoglobin and hemoglobin molecules differ from one species to another, and how this family of oxygen-binding protein chains evolved. In Chapter 4 we shall see what happens when the hemoglobin molecule malfunctions, producing sickle cell anemia and the thalassemias. But first we need a brief introduction to the rules of the game—the nature of a protein as a polymer of amino acids with different side chains, the way in which these side chains differ, and how this affects the folding of the polymer into a three-dimensional, functioning globular molecule. The balance of this chapter should be regarded only as a summary review of some key ideas that will be needed later. More extensive introductions can be found in standard biochemistry texts such as those by Stryer (3), Lehninger (4), or Metzler (5); in *The Structure and Action of Proteins* (6); and in the forthcoming *Proteins: Structure, Function, Evolution* (7). An elementary introduction can be found in reference 8.

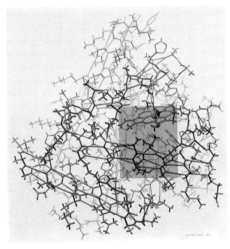

Figure 1.1 Skeletal drawing of the full myoglobin molecule, with the area corresponding to the opening illustration enclosed in a color rectangle. This first full side-chain drawing of any protein molecule was made by Irving Geis in 1961 for *Scientific American*. Some side chains have been identified differently since 1961 in the light of improved x-ray refinement and amino acid analysis. (Drawing based on a model by H. C. Watson, with coordinates courtesy of J. C. Kendrew. Copyright 1961 by *Scientific American*. All rights reserved.)

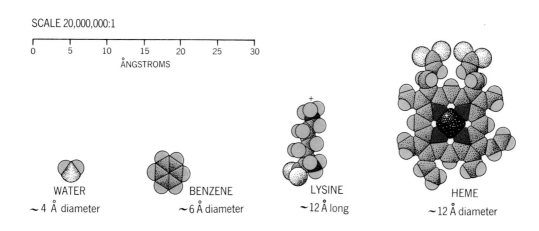

SCALE 20,000,000:1

0   5   10   15   20   25   30
ÅNGSTROMS

WATER
~4 Å diameter

BENZENE
~6 Å diameter

LYSINE
~12 Å long

HEME
~12 Å diameter

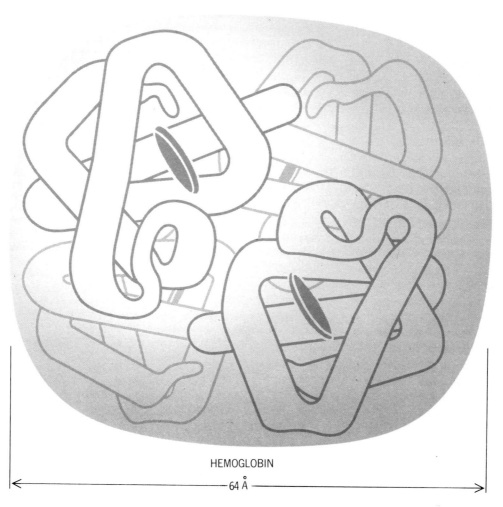

HEMOGLOBIN

$\longleftarrow$ 64 Å $\longrightarrow$

Figure 1.2 Molecular size comparisons. These molecules have all been enlarged by the same linear factor of 20 million times. To appreciate what this means, if you were enlarged by the same factor, the Earth would appear to you as a 2-foot sphere, and your index finger would reach from New York to Kansas City. Molecular dimensions are measured in angstrom units (Å), with 100 million Å to the centimeter or 254 million Å to the inch. Most chemical bonds are between 1 and 3 Å in length.

1.1 PROTEINS AS POLYMERS OF AMINO ACIDS

Figure 1.2 gives an idea of the size of a hemoglobin molecule. Hemoglobin is larger than a water molecule, but it is still a very small object, as can be appreciated by the fact that the molecules shown in Figure 1.2 have been enlarged by 20 million times. The molecular weight of a molecule is the sum of the atomic weights of all the atoms in it, with a hydrogen atom having an atomic weight of 1; carbon, 12; nitrogen, 14; oxygen, 16; sulfur, 32; and iron, 56. Atomic and molecular weights are sometimes given without units, and sometimes assigned units of daltons, after John Dalton, the founder of the atomic theory. There are 602,200,000,000,000,000,000,000 or 6.022×10^{23} daltons in 1 gram. This very large conversion factor between the molecular and the macroscopic worlds is known as Avogadro's number.

Hemoglobin is a reasonably typical protein molecule, with a molecular weight of 64,650. Other proteins range from 5000 to several million. By comparison, a water molecule has a molecular weight of only 18, and benzene, 78. The molecular weight of the smallest amino acid, glycine, is 75, and that of the largest, tryptophan, is 204. The average molecular weight of amino acids in proteins is around 100–110.

An amino acid is so named because it has an NH_2 amine group and a COOH carboxylic acid group on either side of a central carbon atom, which is called the alpha carbon or C_α (Figure 1.3). Also attached to the α carbon are a hydrogen atom and a characteristic side chain, designated by R in Figure 1.3. It is this side chain that makes one amino acid different from another. When two amino acids are connected to form one link in a polypeptide chain, a molecule of water is removed so that the carbon atom of the carboxylic acid group on one amino acid is connected directly to the nitrogen atom of the amine group on the next amino acid. In this way, 100 separate amino acids are turned into a protein chain of 100 amino acid residues. Typical protein chains have 60 to 500 amino acids. The DNA of the genes essentially contains nothing more than a set of instructions specifying the order in which various amino acids must be snapped together to make a particular protein. Once this is done, the folding of the chain into a functional three-dimensional molecule follows without further instructions. Although we know that this is true, we do not yet understand matters well enough to predict, from amino acid sequence alone, how a protein will fold in space. This is one of the most challenging (and frustrating) problems in protein chemistry today.

Two kinds of bonds can make cross-links between loops of the chain: *disulfide bridges* and *hydrogen bonds*. A disulfide bridge is formed when the sulfur atoms of two cysteine residues, which have —CH_2—SH side chains, are connected directly, with the loss of two H atoms, as shown in Figure 1.3. A much more common bridge is the hydrogen bond. This can be formed between a hydrogen atom attached to N or O, and another O atom such as that which is double-bonded to C in the main chain. The bond arises essentially by electrostatic attraction between the slightly positively charged H atom, and one of the two pairs of electrons on oxygen that are not being used in chemical bonding. A single hydrogen bond is weak: around 6 kcal of energy per mole, by comparison with 83 kcal per mole for a carbon–carbon single bond. But hydrogen bonds are important in all biological materials because there are so many of them. They are the threads that stitch protein molecules together.

A protein molecule has the advantage of constructional simplicity that comes from being built from backbone parts of standardized dimensions. The standard bond lengths and angles of a peptide bond in a protein are given in Figure 1.4. Because some of the double-bond character of the C═O bond leaks over into the C─N bond, rotation about that bond is effectively prevented, and all six atoms associated with the colored area in Figure 1.4 are forced to lie in the same plane. This is called the *amide plane*. When amide planes are joined as in Figure 1.5, they are free to rotate about their two bonds to the α carbon that connects them. Rotations of the backbone amides direct the protein chain toward its final three-dimensional conformation, and the fact that there are only two such rotations per amino acid residue is an important limit on possible protein folding.

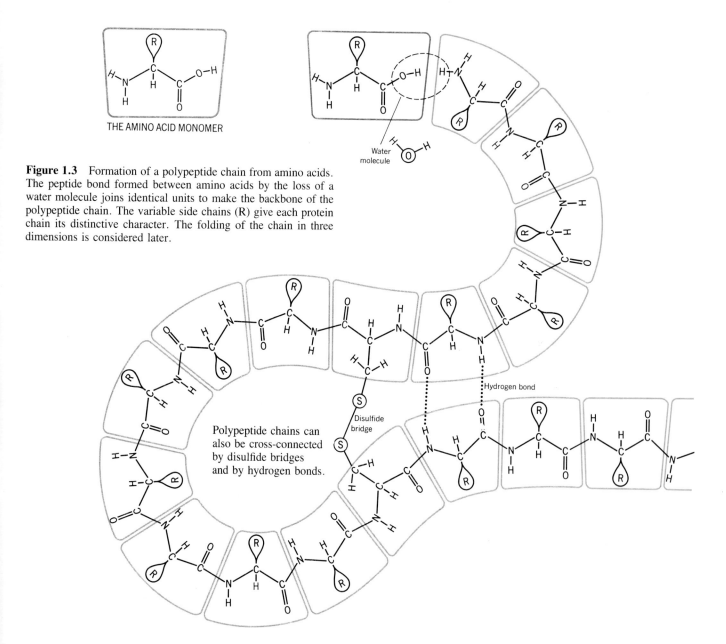

THE AMINO ACID MONOMER

Figure 1.3 Formation of a polypeptide chain from amino acids. The peptide bond formed between amino acids by the loss of a water molecule joins identical units to make the backbone of the polypeptide chain. The variable side chains (R) give each protein chain its distinctive character. The folding of the chain in three dimensions is considered later.

Water molecule

Polypeptide chains can also be cross-connected by disulfide bridges and by hydrogen bonds.

Disulfide bridge

Hydrogen bond

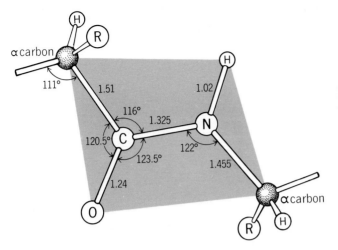

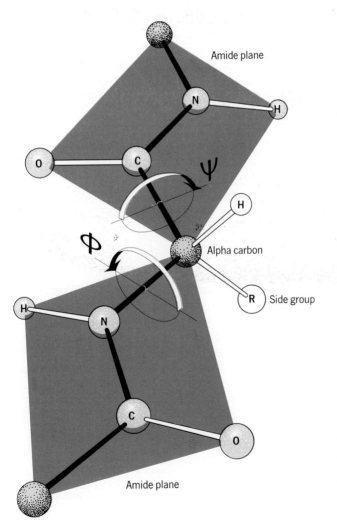

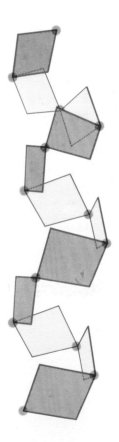

Figure 1.4 Geometry of the polypeptide bond. The partial double-bond character of the C — N bond means that all of the atoms connected by the colored quadrilateral lie in the same plane, called the amide plane or polypeptide plane. This restriction is important in defining the folding of a protein in three dimensions. (Distances in angstroms.)

Figure 1.5 Two amide planes joined by the tetrahedral bonds of the α carbon. The only possible rotation of the main chain is that about the C_α — C bond (designated by ψ) and the C_α — N bond (designated by ϕ). These amide planes, connected at opposite corners by C_α atoms (gray dots), define the polypeptide backbone, shown here in a helical conformation.

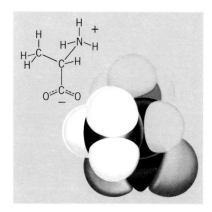
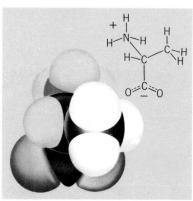

Figure 1.6 L-Alanine and its enantiomorph (mirror image), D-alanine. The skeletal drawings are easier to understand, but the space-filling drawings depicting atoms as interconnected spheres give a more accurate impression of the appearance of an amino acid molecule.

The four groups connected to an α carbon of a protein—amine group, carboxylic acid, hydrogen, and side chain—are directed toward the four corners of a tetrahedron, with the α carbon in the center. As with any atom having a tetrahedral arrangement of four different groups, the attachment can be made in two different ways, related by mirror reflection like right and left hands. These are differentiated by calling them L (for *levulo,* "left") and D (for *dextro,* "right") enantiomorphs of the amino acids. The two mirror enantiomorphs of the amino acid alanine are compared in Figure 1.6. Although one form is no more and no less likely than the other in isolation, the amino acids of living organisms on Earth do not exist in isolation: They are made and manipulated by enzymes, which themselves are proteins built from amino acids. Life on this planet is based only on L-amino acids. Although we can see no intrinsic advantage of one form over the other, there is an advantage of simplicity, for enzymatic reactions, in having only one form. Unless there is more to the problem than we now realize, life on another planet would have a 50:50 chance of being based on D- or L-amino acids (assuming that it had evolved along similar lines to our own life but independently from it). Nevertheless, the choice was made once on Earth, and has been adhered to ever since: L-amino acids only. The geometry of an L-amino acid is easy to remember with the mnemonic trick sketched in Figure 1.7.

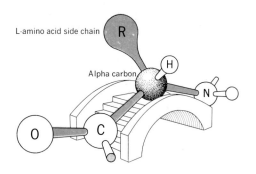

Figure 1.7 The stereochemistry of L- and D-amino acids can be remembered by imagining the backbone at the α carbon as an arched bridge to be crossed from CO to N (remember carbON or ONward). The side chain of L-amino acids then extends to the left, and that of D-amino acids to the right.

1.2 THE VARIETY OF AMINO ACIDS

Although the number of possible amino acids with different side chains is endless, the genetic code of all living organisms on Earth is restricted to a set of 20 amino acids, whose side chains are depicted in Figure 1.8. The way in which these side chains are attached to the main polypeptide chain is shown in Figure 1.9. At first the variety of side chains may appear meaningless and confusing, but with examination a pattern begins to emerge. Four side chains are hydrocarbons (valine, leucine, isoleucine, phenylalanine) of different sizes and shapes. These are hydrophobic or "water-hating" side chains, and prefer to remain buried on the inside of a globular protein molecule, away from the aqueous environment of the cell. For this reason they are classified in Figure 1.8 as *internal* amino acids. A fifth, methionine, is counted as a member of this group because its —S—sulfur atom within the hydrocarbon chain acts like a —CH$_2$— group.

Figure 1.8 The 20 genetically coded amino acids. Only the side chains are shown, and these are grouped into three categories: *external*→ (polar and charged side chains), *internal* (generally nonpolar), and *ambivalent* (capable of occurring inside or outside a folded protein molecule). Each of the 20 amino acids is designated by its name, its three-letter code, and its one-letter code in parentheses. The forms shown here are those prevalent at pH 7 (neutrality): Aspartic and glutamic acids are ionized and negatively charged, lysine and arginine are protonated and positively charged, and histidine is 50% uncharged (shown here) and 50% protonated and positively charged.

EXTERNAL

ACIDIC

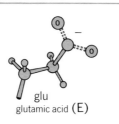

asp
aspartic acid (D)

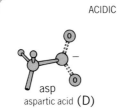

glu
glutamic acid (E)

BASIC

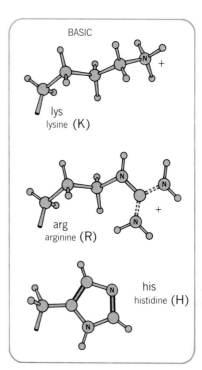

lys
lysine (K)

arg
arginine (R)

his
histidine (H)

NEUTRAL

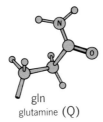

asn
asparagine (N)

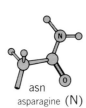

gln
glutamine (Q)

Asparagine and glutamine, although neutral, have very polar side chains that cause them to be generally on the outside of the molecule. In these side chain drawings, heavy double lines indicate double bonds, and dashed lines indicate resonance bonds intermediate between single and double bonds.

AMBIVALENT

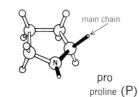

main chain

pro
proline (P)

thr
threonine (T)

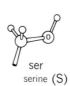

ser
serine (S)

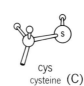

cys
cysteine (C)

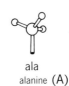

ala
alanine (A)

gly
glycine (G)

INTERNAL

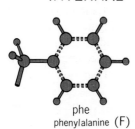

tyr
tyrosine (Y)

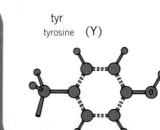

trp
tryptophan (W)

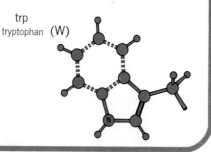

phe
phenylalanine (F)

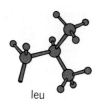

leu
leucine (L)

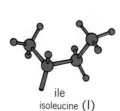

ile
isoleucine (I)

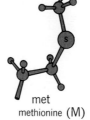

met
methionine (M)

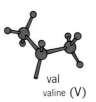

val
valine (V)

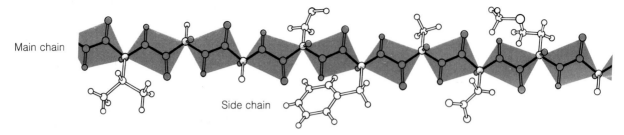

Main chain

Side chain

Figure 1.9 The amide link (CO—NH) is the repeating unit of the main chain; the side chains vary.

In contrast to these, seven amino acids are classified as *external* because they are so polar, or even charged, that they prefer an aqueous environment on the outside of a protein. Of these, aspartic and glutamic acids have carboxylic acid groups (Figure 1.10a), which at neutral pH are ionized with the loss of a proton (a hydrogen ion, H^+), giving the side chains a negative charge. The amide derivatives of these two, asparagine and glutamine, have no negative charge. But they are so polar that they are almost always encountered on the surface of protein molecules. Three other external side chains are organic bases: Lysine has an amine group (Figure 1.10b), arginine has a more extended guanidino group (Figure 1.10c), and histidine has an imidazole ring (Figure 1.10d). These three have nitrogen atoms with unused electron pairs that can attract protons, resulting in a positive charge on the side chain. At the neutral conditions found in a cell, lysines and arginines are completely protonated and positively charged, and histidines are roughly 50% charged (right in Figure 1.10d) and 50% uncharged (left in Figure 1.10d).

A final eight amino acid side chains are neither so hydrophobic that they are forced to remain inside, nor so polar that they must remain outside. These are the *ambivalent* residues; perhaps "indifferent" might be a better term. Glycine has only a hydrogen atom for its side chain, and is particularly useful in tight corners in the interior of a protein where there is no room for a bulkier group. Alanine, technically, has a hydrocarbon side chain, but the CH_3 group is so small that a negligible price in energy is paid in bringing it out to the surface of a protein molecule. Cysteine, serine, and threonine are polar, but only moderately so, and can tolerate being inside a protein molecule, especially if the OH group of serine or threonine is involved in a hydrogen bond to another atom. Tyrosine and tryptophan, although built from aromatic rings like the hydrophobic phenylalanine, have polar OH and NH groups on their rings that can be used in hydrogen bonding. Cysteine, as was mentioned earlier, can join sulfur atoms with a second cysteine to build a disulfide bridge between two chains. Proline is the odd amino acid out, in that its side chain from the α carbon loops back to make a second connection to its amine nitrogen. This forces a contorted bend on the main polypeptide chain. Prolines are especially useful in reversing the direction of a chain that is heading out from the center of a globular protein, and sending it back toward the interior again. For this reason, prolines are frequently encountered at the surface of protein molecules, even though they technically have hydrocarbon side chains and hence might have been classified among the internal amino acids.

Hydrogen bonds are the lacing that stitches a protein molecule together. Figure 1.3 shows the most common kind, between the NH and CO of the main polypeptide chain. But the NH or NH_2 of asparagine, glutamine, lysine, arginine, histidine, and tryptophan can also act as hydrogen atom donors in such a

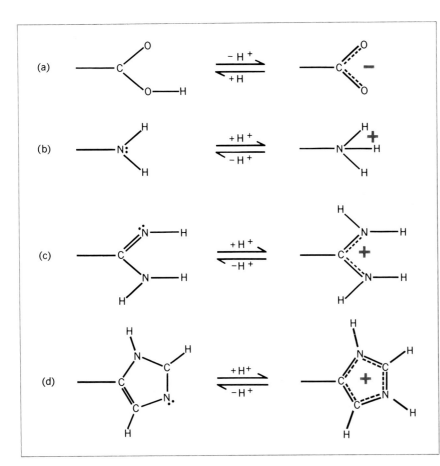

Figure 1.10 Acidic and basic groups found in protein side chains. Aspartic and glutamic acids contain the carboxyl group (a), which can lose a hydrogen atom or proton and acquire a negative charge. Lysine side chains have an amine group (b), whose nitrogen electron pair can attract a proton and hence acquire a positive charge. Arginine has a more complicated guanidino group (c), but the principle of acquiring an H^+ ion is the same. Histidine (d) can attract a proton to one of its imidazole ring nitrogens. Dashed lines in these drawings represent electrons that are shared or delocalized among several atoms, lowering the overall energy of the group and making it more stable.

bond (Figure 1.11a, b), as can the OH groups of serine, threonine, and tyrosine (Figure 1.11c, d). The oxygen atoms of these OH groups can also function as hydrogen-bond acceptors, as can the CO of asparagine and glutamine. All of these groups are polar, and therefore energetically unhappy in the hydrophobic interior of a protein molecule. But their combination into a hydrogen bond represents a kind of neutralization—whenever these groups occur inside a protein, they are almost always paired off in hydrogen bonds. One of the best ways of gently unfolding a globular protein molecule is to place it in a solution of urea, $H_2N—CO—NH_2$. This molecule can act as both donor and acceptor for hydrogen bonding. It encourages a protein to unfold and replace many of its internal hydrogen bonds with new bonds to urea molecules. If the urea then is removed gently by dialysis or other means, the protein can be induced to refold into its original structure. This, incidentally, is one of the most convincing experimental proofs that the amino acid sequence of a protein contains all the information needed for self-assembly, without the necessity of any kind of template enzymes. Hence the three-dimensional structure of a protein molecule can be reduced logically to a one-dimensional sequence of amino acids or ultimately of bases in the DNA of the gene for the proteins, which makes the problem of information storage in the genes far simpler.

The hydrogen atom in a hydrogen bond is attracted to an unused electron pair on the acceptor nitrogen or oxygen. But atoms having such electron pairs can also attract metal ions, and when they do so they are said to be serving as metal *ligands*. The histidine side chain is an especially common ligand to iron and other metal atoms, and this is how the heme group is held in place in hemoglobin. In other proteins, the sulfur atom of methionine or the oxygen atom of aspartic acid, glutamic acid, asparagine, or glutamine is found as a ligand

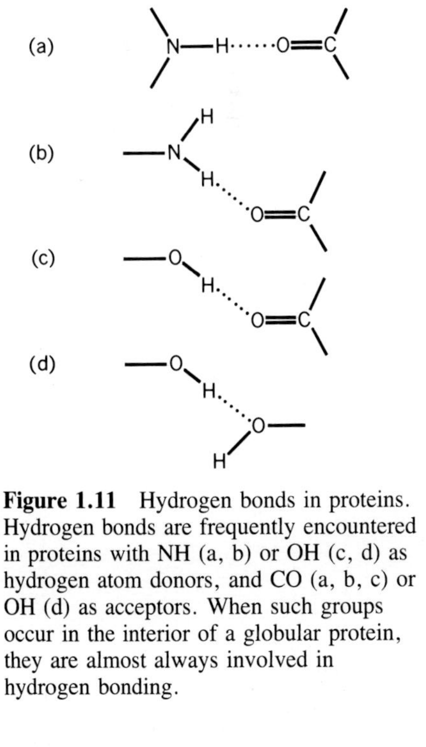

Figure 1.11 Hydrogen bonds in proteins. Hydrogen bonds are frequently encountered in proteins with NH (a, b) or OH (c, d) as hydrogen atom donors, and CO (a, b, c) or OH (d) as acceptors. When such groups occur in the interior of a globular protein, they are almost always involved in hydrogen bonding.

to iron, zinc, copper, or other metals. This may be why methionine, with side chain $—CH_2—CH_2—S—CH_3$, is one of the 20 genetically coded amino acids used today whereas its purely hydrocarbon analog norleucine, $—CH_2—CH_2—CH_2—CH_3$, is not. Methionine can function as well as norleucine can as an internal residue, and has the additional ability to act as a metal ligand. It would be a loss to replace methionine by norleucine in the genetic code, and wasteful to carry them both. This probably is one example of the way in which the genetic code itself is the consequence of natural selection early in the history of life.

In summary, the 20 amino acid side chains that are specified today by the genetic code have a wide variety of properties. Some are very polar, and others are hydrophobic, thus influencing the regions of chain in which they occur to fold on the outside or the inside of a globular protein molecule. Many can form hydrogen bonds, which help to lace up the interior of the molecule. Some can hold on to metal atoms, and one, cysteine, can make a direct covalent bond from one protein chain to another. The acidic and basic side chains anchor negative and positive charges on the molecular surface, and these can be useful in enzymatic catalysis and in the recognition of one protein molecule by another. The tool kit of side chains in Figure 1.8 seems too haphazard to be the result of rational design, but too orderly to be random. It most probably is the result of a long period of trial and error, starting with the spectrum of prebiotic amino acids that was available in the Earth's oceans when life first evolved.

1.3 THE FOLDING OF A PROTEIN CHAIN

Architects learned long ago that it is easier to build a complex structure if its construction is modular—that is, if it is built from smaller units of standard size and shape. Bricks are one such standard module, as are wooden two-by-fours, even if they are not two-by-four anything by the time they reach the users' hands. (They are almost exactly 4×8 cm, however, which promises a fine confusion in nomenclature if the United States ever bestirs itself and joins the rest of the world in using the metric system.) The linear polypeptide chain in proteins frequently is found to be organized into two distinctive modular structures, which then are packed together to build the entire protein molecule. These modules are the α helix and the β sheet.

The α helix is the central helix in Figure 1.12. The successive turns of the helix are held together by hydrogen bonds from one turn to the next. If the acceptor is the $C=O$ of amino acid residue n (numbering, as always, from the end with the free NH_2 amine group to the end with the free COOH carboxyl group), then the donor is the NH of residue $n + 4$, farther along the chain. The α helix has 3.6 amino acid residues per turn of helix. It is a particularly unstrained structure, and is one of the commonest features of proteins. If the CO of residue n is bonded instead to the NH of residue $n + 3$, the result is the more tightly wound 3_{10} helix, and if it is bonded to residue $n + 5$, the looser π helix results (left and right in Figure 1.12a). Each of these is less stable than the α helix. Occasional stretches of 3_{10} helix are seen, but a complete π helix by itself has never been found in proteins. A more common behavior is for the final turn of an α helix to be tightened up to the hydrogen-bonding pattern of one turn of 3_{10} helix, or unwrapped like a final turn of π. Hemoglobin and myoglobin are essentially constructed from packed α helices, many of them capped off by a turn of 3_{10} or π. The α helix is also the basic building block of fibrous proteins such as hair, wool, and muscle fibers.

(a)

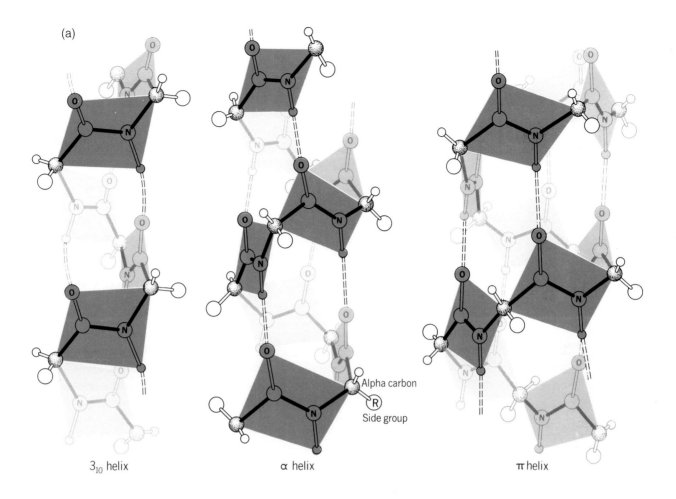

3_{10} helix α helix π helix

Alpha carbon
Side group

(b)

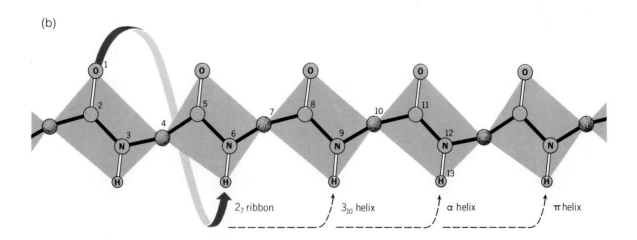

2_7 ribbon 3_{10} helix α helix π helix

Figure 1.12 Coiling of polypeptide chains into helices. (a) The 3_{10}, α, and π helices differ in their patterns of hydrogen bonding, shown in (b). Hydrogen bonds in the α helix are particularly unstrained, making the α helix especially stable. The α carbons are stippled, with small attached spheres for hydrogens and larger spheres for side chains. (b) Hydrogen-bonding pattern from one turn of the helix to the next, for four related helices. Only the α helix is found extensively in proteins; the others are found only occasionally for very short stretches, usually winding down or unwinding the last turn of an α helix.

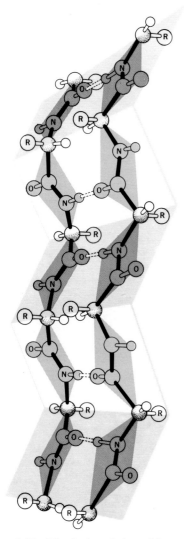

The β sheet is formed when several polypeptide chains are laid down next to one another, either parallel or antiparallel, and then cross-connected by CO···HN hydrogen bonds at right angles to the chain direction, as in Figure 1.13. That drawing shows only two chains, but more could be added to the left and right. Because such sheets tend to form corrugations or pleats that push the side chains out as far as possible away from the sheet surface, they are called β *pleated sheets*. Such sheets are the basic structure of silk fibers. The protein chains themselves lie parallel to the fiber direction and make the fibers tough and hard to break. Also, the ability of stacks of sheets to slide over one another like pages in a book makes silk fibers flexible and supple. The β sheet is not found in hemoglobin or myoglobin, but is the central organizing unit in many enzymes and other proteins.

The Danish biochemist K. Linderstrøm-Lang proposed in 1952, long before any protein structures actually were known, that such structures would be modular in nature. He defined the order of amino acid residues along the unfolded protein chain as the *primary* structure, the folding of this chain into local features such as helices and sheets as the *secondary* structure, and the packing of these helices and sheets against one another to build the complete three-dimensional molecule as the *tertiary* structure (Figure 1.14). This terminology is universally used today, with the addition of *quaternary* structure to designate the way in which independent subunits such as the four chains of hemoglobin are arranged relative to one another (Figure 1.15). So far, in this introductory chapter, we have considered the primary and secondary structures of proteins. Now we want to turn to higher levels of organization of the hemoglobin family of proteins. We shall see how, in the words of the great architect and inventor of the modern skyscraper, Louis H. Sullivan, "Form follows function." We shall also see how, in a more immediate sense, function follows form. In short, what is the molecular basis for the behavior of hemoglobin?

Figure 1.13 The β pleated sheet. Many roughly parallel polypeptide chains can be connected by lateral hydrogen bonds to form an extended sheet structure. It folds naturally into pleats or ridges, with the side chains, — R, pointing out on either side. The individual strands of the sheet can run in opposite directions (antiparallel β sheet), the same direction (parallel β sheet), or a mixture of the two.

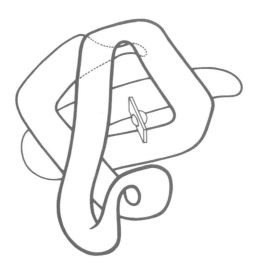

Figure 1.14 Tertiary structure as seen in a single polypeptide chain of a beta subunit (monomer) of hemoglobin.

GENERAL REFERENCES

1. Barcroft, J., 1928. *The Respiratory Function of the Blood*, Cambridge University Press, Cambridge, p.1.
2. Reichert, E. T., and Brown, A. P., 1909. *The Crystallography of the Hemoglobins*, Carnegie Institute of Washington, Washington, D.C.
3. Stryer, L., 1981. *Biochemistry* (2nd ed.), Freeman, San Francisco.
4. Lehninger, A. L., 1982. *Principles of Biochemistry*, Worth, New York.
5. Metzler, D. E., 1977. *Biochemistry*, Academic Press, New York.
6. Dickerson, R. E., and Geis, I., 1969. *The Structure and Action of Proteins*, Benjamin/Cummings, Menlo Park.
7. Dickerson, R. E., and Geis, I., in preparation. *Proteins: Structure, Function, Evolution*, Benjamin/Cummings, Menlo Park.
8. Dickerson, R. E., and Geis, I., 1976. *Chemistry, Matter, and the Universe*, Benjamin/Cummings, Menlo Park.

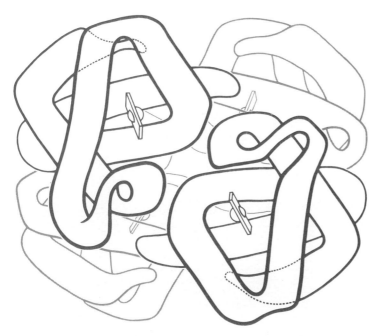

Figure 1.15 Quaternary structure as seen in the arrangement of the four subunits of the functioning hemoglobin tetramer.

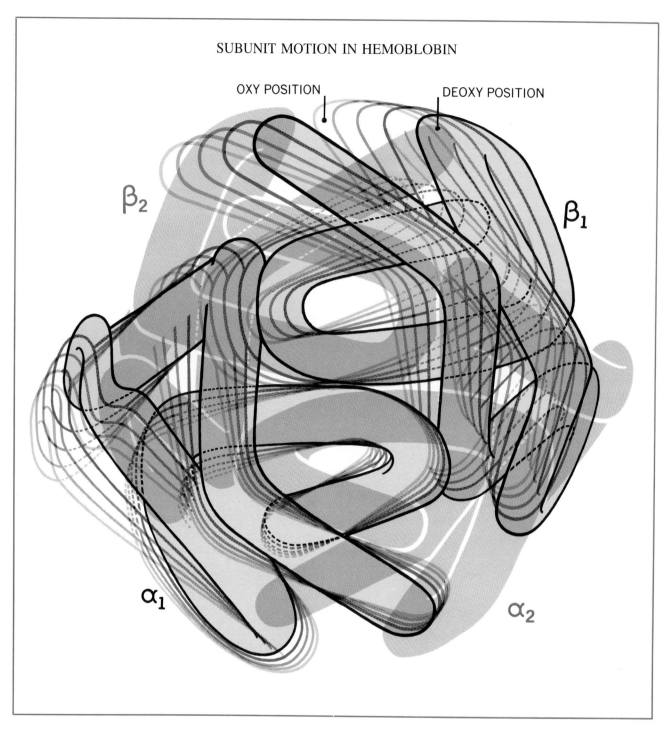

SUBUNIT MOTION IN HEMOBLOBIN

OXY POSITION   DEOXY POSITION

β_2 β_1

α_1 α_2

The fanciful "stroboscopic" hemoglobin above illustrates the ability of the molecule to respond to changes in its environment. Oxyhemoglobin (R conformation) is one of the extreme states of the tetramer. It is ideally suited to binding oxygen in the lungs, where oxygen is plentiful. The other extreme state, deoxyhemoglobin (T conformation) allows oxygen to be readily released in the tissues where oxygen tension is lower. The first oxygen bound to a heme iron facilitates the binding of subsequent oxygens. Like-wise, when fully oxygenated hemoglobin drops its first oxygen, others are more easily released. This effect is not seen in monomers or dimers. Only the tetramer with its transition between R and T states exhibits "cooperativity." The change in conformation is mediated by H^+, CO_2, Cl^-, and DPG—all of which bind preferentially to de-oxyhemoglobin and encourage the tetramer to release its oxygen cargo. In the drawing above, the $\alpha_1\beta_1$ dimer in black is shown moving relative to the $\alpha_2\beta_2$ dimer, in color.

2 HEMOGLOBIN STRUCTURE AND FUNCTION

CHAPTER TWO

HEMOGLOBIN STRUCTURE AND FUNCTION

Hemoglobin, the oxygen carrier of the blood, is the one protein molecule that everyone knows. Myoglobin, the oxygen-storage protein of muscle, is less familiar. They were the first proteins whose structures were worked out by x-ray crystallography. They were also among the first to have their amino acid sequences determined. Most of the basic concepts of molecular evolution really began with the globin structures and sequences, and more comparative sequence information is available today for the globins than for any other protein except cytochrome *c*. High-resolution structure refinements of various forms of the globins make them a case study of the way in which structural information can explain the chemical properties of a protein molecule. If we were to go into the history of the changing theories of how the hemoglobin molecule functions (which we shall not), that history would provide a classic example of the way that protein structures suggest mechanistic theories and models, which in turn suggest new chemical experiments, whose results provide feedback that forces the original theories to be abandoned, modified, qualified, and improved until the truth is finally approached asymptotically. This chapter is concerned with the structure and properties of the vertebrate globins; the next chapter introduces their evolutionary history, and the final chapter deals with abnormal human hemoglobins.

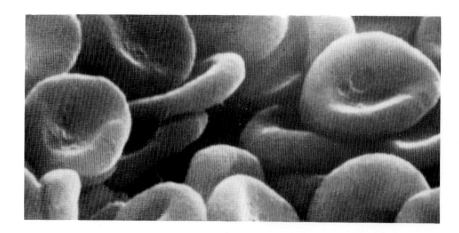

Figure 2.1 Scanning electron micrograph of human red blood cells. Normal red cells are a relatively constant 7.5 microns in diameter. (Photo courtesy Dr. Thomas Hayes, Lawrence Livermore National Laboratory.)

Hemoglobin and its cousin myoglobin are two of the most important and plentiful proteins of vertebrates. Every milliliter of blood has approximately 5 billion erythrocytes or red cells (Figure 2.1), and each erythrocyte is packed with 280 million molecules of hemoglobin.* A molecule of hemoglobin has four heme groups, each associated with a protein chain of molecular weight around 16,000. The muscle protein that gives good steak its red color is not hemoglobin, but myoglobin. It has one heme group and one protein chain, of about the same size as each of the four hemoglobin chains. The role of hemoglobin is to bind molecular oxygen to its heme irons at the lungs and to deliver it to the tissues; that of myoglobin in voluntary muscle is to store oxygen until it is required for metabolic oxidation. A second task of hemoglobin is to bring the carbon dioxide by-product of oxidation back to the lungs to get rid of it (1–5).†

Binding to hemoglobin is not the only way oxygen can be transported by the blood; some O_2 dissolves directly in the plasma, but the solubility of oxygen gas in blood plasma is directly proportional to the partial pressure of O_2 in contact with the plasma. At the 100-mm oxygen pressure found in the lungs, only 0.3 mL of oxygen gas can dissolve per 100 mL of plasma, far too little to keep a human being going. One would have to breathe pure O_2 at 3 atm pressure for the solubility to rise to an acceptable 7 mL oxygen per 100 mL plasma, and this would be sufficient only for someone sitting quietly at rest. In contrast, the 15 g of hemoglobin found in 100 mL of normal human blood are capable of binding 20 mL of gaseous O_2 if the hemoglobin molecules are fully saturated. The actual degree of saturation varies with oxygen partial pressure, but, as we shall see shortly, the saturation of hemoglobin as it passes through the lungs is almost complete.

The heart of both hemoglobin and myoglobin is the heme group, an iron atom surrounded by a porphyrin ring (Figure 2.2). The porphyrin ring is unsaturated in the same sense that benzene is unsaturated, and has many delocalized π electrons. Only one of many possible resonance bond structures, or combinations of single and double bonds, is shown in the figure. The backbone actually has cloverleaf symmetry, with bonds *a* and *a'*, *b* and *b'*, *c* and *c'*, and *d* and *d'* being equivalent. Surrounding the heme in sperm whale myoglobin is a protein or polypeptide chain with 153 amino acids and a molecular weight of 17,199 (Figure 2.3). The human hemoglobin molecule has a total of four chains—two identical chains labeled α, with 141 amino acids and 15,126 molecular weight, and two identical β chains, with 146 residues and 15,867 molecular weight each. The heme adds another 616 daltons to each chain, so the total molecular weight of sperm whale myoglobin is 17,815, and that of the human hemoglobin tetramer is 64,450. The four-chain structure of hemoglobin is directly related to the way it behaves in fulfilling its biological role.

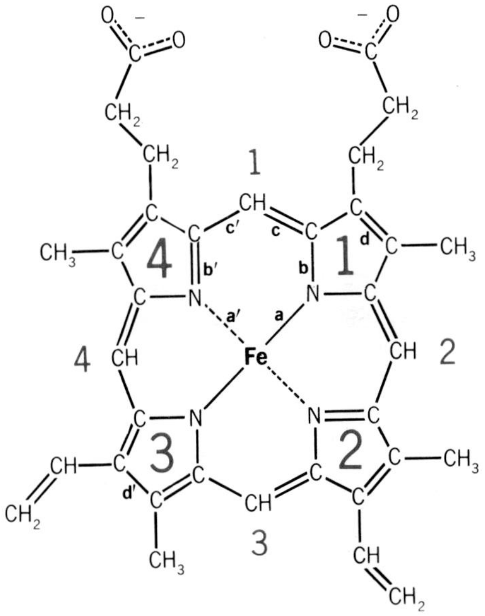

Figure 2.2 The heme group is an essential component in hemoglobins, cytochromes, and enzymes such as catalase and peroxidase. The central porphyrin ring has various side chains: methyl, —CH_3; vinyl, —CH=CH_2; and propionic acid, —CH_2—CH_2—COOH. The numbering of five-membered rings and bridging —CH— will be useful later for identification purposes.

---

*If an erythrocyte were enlarged 300 million times, it would be the size, and roughly the shape, of the Rose Bowl, piled high with 280 million large grapefruit.

†At the end of each chapter is a list of general references, which are identified within the chapter by their numbers. Hence (1–5) indicates the first five general references. Following this list is an Appendix listing all the relevant x-ray analyses of proteins that have been carried out to date. This Appendix has its own list of references, which are identified within the chapter by an "A" before the reference number. Hence (A15) indicates reference 15 of the Appendix reference list.

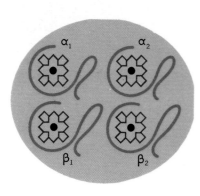

Figure 2.3 (a) Myoglobin is built from one heme group and a polypeptide chain of 153 amino acids. (b) Hemoglobin has four hemes and four polypeptide chains, two α with 141 amino acids, and two β with 146.

The hemoglobin/myoglobin pair has not always been the answer to the problem of distributing oxygen. One-celled organisms and creatures up to about 1 mm across can distribute oxygen by simple molecular diffusion. Many invertebrates have globins, but others use nonheme metalloproteins instead. Insects have surmounted the size barrier by developing hollow tracheal tubes, and can remain dependent upon gaseous diffusion. But this will work only up to a point. As J. B. S. Haldane has pointed out, this is one of the main reasons that insects have remained small—and why the horror-film stories of giant man-eating ants are unlikely to come true.

Myoglobin and hemoglobin are excellent examples of molecular "engineering"—the fine-tuning of molecular properties for the tasks at hand. The properties that are desirable in an oxygen-transporting system can be summarized as follows:

1. The carrier (hemoglobin) should have a high affinity for oxygen in the presence of a plentiful supply at the lungs, and a lowered affinity in the oxygen-poorer environment of the muscles.

2. The storage molecule (myoglobin) should have a higher affinity for oxygen than the carrier has at low oxygen concentrations.

3. The carrier should be able to transport carbon dioxide back to the lungs where it can be ejected as a waste product.

4. The carrier should release its oxygen more readily to working muscle, with its buildup of lactic acid and of carbonic acid from CO_2, than to resting muscle, which needs less oxygen.

The two globins show all of these properties, as illustrated in Figure 2.4. Most of these properties are also implicit in the saturation curves in Figure 2.5. The oxygen-binding curve for myoglobin (Mb) is the hyperbola expected for the simple one-to-one association of myoglobin heme and oxygen:

$$\text{Mb} + O_2 \rightleftarrows \text{MbO}_2 \qquad A = \frac{[\text{MbO}_2]}{[\text{Mb}][O_2]} = \text{equilibrium association constant*}$$

Brackets around a substance, as in $[\text{MbO}_2]$, represent the concentration of the substance. If y is the fraction of myoglobin molecules saturated and if the oxygen concentration is expressed in terms of the partial pressure of oxygen, P_{O_2}, then

$$A = \frac{y}{(1-y)P_{O_2}} \qquad \text{and} \qquad y = \frac{AP_{O_2}}{1 + AP_{O_2}}$$

This is the equation of the hyperbola labeled "myoglobin" in Figure 2.5.

Hemoglobin (Hb) behaves differently. Its S-shaped (or sigmoid) curve requires an overall association constant expression with a greater-than-first-power dependence upon the oxygen concentration. The following expression, known as the *Hill equation,* fits the middle part of the oxygen equilibrium curve well:

$$A = \frac{[\text{HbO}_2]}{[\text{Hb}][O_2]^n} \qquad \text{and} \qquad y = \frac{AP_{O_2}^n}{1 + AP_{O_2}^n}$$

---

*We shall use A for association constant to avoid confusion with the conventional K for dissociation constant. $A = 1/K$.

The exponent n, called the *Hill coefficient,* is observed to be around 2.8 rather than 1.0, as for myoglobin. This indicates that the binding of oxygen molecules to the four hemes is not independent; binding to any one heme is affected by the state of the other three. The first oxygen attaches itself very weakly to the heme. It has a low association constant, A_1, of 5–60 atm^{-1}, depending on pH and concentrations of chloride, CO_2, and the organophosphate molecule 2,3-diphosphoglycerate or DPG (values from reference A25 and sources quoted therein):

$$\text{Hb} + O_2 \rightleftarrows \text{HbO}_2 \qquad A_1 = \frac{[\text{HbO}_2]}{[\text{Hb}][O_2]} = 5 - 60 \text{ atm}^{-1}$$

The second and third oxygens then bind more strongly, and the last oxygen has two to three orders of magnitude greater affinity than the first oxygen:

$$\text{Hb} \cdot 3O_2 + O_2 \rightleftarrows \text{Hb} \cdot 4O_2 \qquad A_4 = \frac{[\text{Hb} \cdot 4O_2]}{[\text{Hb} \cdot 3O_2][O_2]} = 3000 - 6000 \text{ atm}^{-1}$$

The last heme to bind oxygen in hemoglobin does so somewhat better than myoglobin ($A_M = 1500$ atm^{-1}) or isolated hemoglobin subunits do ($A_\alpha = 1500$ atm^{-1}; $A_\beta = 2600$ atm^{-1}). (All of these constants were measured at 25°C. Since the reaction with oxygen is exothermic or heat emitting, the oxygen affinity decreases with rising temperature.) Hence the four-chain hemoglobin tetramer functions, not by enhancing the binding of the last oxygen molecules, but by diminishing the tendency to bind the first ones. When a fully loaded hemoglobin molecule arrives at the tissues, its tendency to keep or lose the first oxygen is about the same as that of myoglobin. But with each oxygen lost, the next one falls off more easily. The hemoglobin molecule behaves as an all-or-nothing oxygen carrier, in what Max Perutz has called the *Matthew effect:* "For to him who has will more be given, and he will have abundance; but from him who has not, even that which he has shall be taken away" (Matt. 13:12). Most hemoglobin molecules are found with either no oxygen (*deoxyhemoglobin*) or four oxygens (*oxyhemoglobin*). The intermediate oxygenation states are present in much lower concentrations.

The deoxyhemoglobin molecule has a higher affinity for protons than does oxyhemoglobin. Hence under acid conditions, with an excess of protons present, the equilibrium between deoxy- and oxyhemoglobin is shifted in favor of deoxyhemoglobin. This equilibrium can be written symbolically, without worrying about the number of protons or oxygen molecules involved, as follows:

$$\underset{\text{oxy}}{\text{HbO}_2} + H^+ \rightleftarrows \underset{\text{deoxy}}{\text{HbH}^+} + O_2$$

Protons and oxygen molecules here are antagonists. When one binds to hemoglobin, the other falls away. The consequence is that the oxygen-saturation curve for hemoglobin is shifted toward the right with increasing acidity (Figure 2.5). This is known as the *Bohr effect,* and is physiologically useful since oxygen has the greatest tendency to dissociate from hemoglobin just when muscle acidity indicates that it is most needed.

Three other naturally occurring substances are known to encourage human oxyhemoglobin to drop its cargo: carbon dioxide, chloride ions, and DPG (Figure 2.6). Carbon dioxide exerts its effect in part by producing protons when it dissolves in blood plasma to form bicarbonate ions:

$$CO_2 + H_2O \rightarrow HCO_3^- + H^+$$

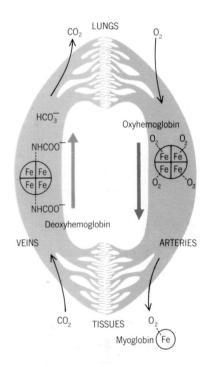

Figure 2.4 Oxygen is carried from the lungs to the tissues by hemoglobin, and carbon dioxide is carried back to the lungs. Part of the CO_2 transport occurs because the amino termini of the four chains in hemoglobin can bind CO_2 directly to form carbamino compounds:

$$R—NH_2 + CO_2 \rightarrow$$
$$R—NH—COO^- + H^+$$

Another factor is the simple buffering ability of the deoxyhemoglobin molecules, which can combine with protons and aid the formation of bicarbonate ions from CO_2 in the blood plasma:

$$CO_2 + H_2O \rightarrow HCO_3^- + H^+$$

The protons are picked up by hemoglobin as it drops its O_2, and the bicarbonate ions are carried back to the lungs in the blood along with deoxyhemoglobin. When the hemoglobin is reoxygenated at the lungs, it releases protons. These protons shift the CO_2 equilibrium just shown to the left, converting bicarbonate ions to the less soluble CO_2, which is exhaled.

Carbon dioxide, chloride ions, and DPG also exert an effect because each binds to deoxyhemoglobin better than to oxyhemoglobin, shifting the equilibrium in favor of the release of oxygen. Carbon dioxide forms carbamates with the amino group at the beginning of each hemoglobin chain,

$$-NH_2 + CO_2 \rightarrow -NH-COO^- + H^+$$

although why this should be possible with deoxyhemoglobin and not with oxyhemoglobin requires explanation, as do the preferences of protons, chloride, and DPG for the unoxygenated molecules.

Protons and carbon dioxide are short-term feedback-control agents. When an oxygen shortage causes lactic acid to build up, or when a very active metabolism leads to high concentrations of carbon dioxide, then the hemoglobin molecules are stimulated to release O_2 more easily. DPG is also a feedback effector on a somewhat longer time scale. Each human red blood cell has approximately as many DPG molecules as it has hemoglobin molecules, and neither can escape through the cell membrane. DPG normally assists hemoglobin in unloading its oxygen. But if oxygen is in chronically short supply, the body is stimulated to synthesize extra quantities of DPG, forcing hemoglobin to drop its O_2 more readily. Bolivians who live at 15,000 ft in the Andes have 20% higher levels of DPG in their red blood cells than do people who live at sea level. (They also have more red blood cells, and hence more hemoglobin, per cubic centimeter of blood.)

The fine-tuning of oxygen affinity by DPG that humans have is found in some other mammals: most primates, marsupials, horses, camels, dogs, pigs, and rodents. In other mammals, such as cattle, sheep, goats, deer, cats, and even one primate, the lemur, the hemoglobin molecule has a smaller oxygen affinity to begin with, and is relatively unaffected by DPG. In birds the regulatory function of DPG is taken over by a similar organophosphate molecule, inositol pentaphosphate (IPP).

In the fetus before birth an additional transfer of oxygen has to take place—from the blood of the mother to that of the fetus. This means that the hemoglobin of the fetus ideally should bind oxygen at concentrations sufficiently

(a)

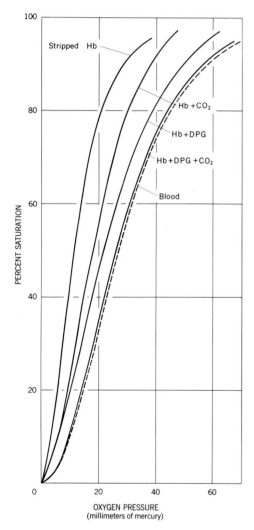

(b)

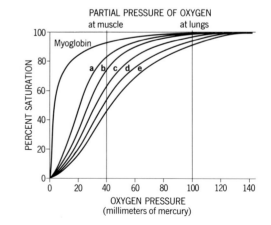

Figure 2.5 Oxygen-binding curves for myoglobin and hemoglobin. (a) Hemoglobin binding curves under various conditions. From left to right: stripped hemoglobin, hemoglobin plus CO_2, hemoglobin plus DPG, hemoglobin plus both CO_2 and DPG, and whole blood (dashed). (b) Myoglobin, and hemoglobin at five different pH values: *a*, 7.6; *b*, 7.4; *c*, 7.2; *d*, 7.0; and *e*, 6.8. The change of oxygen affinity with pH is known as the Bohr effect. Figure 2.5a from Reference 15.

low that the maternal hemoglobin gives up its oxygen. Normal adult $\alpha_2\beta_2$ tetrameric hemoglobin is called *hemoglobin A*. Human fetal hemoglobin, called *hemoglobin F*, has the two α chains of the adult, but its β chains are replaced by similar but not identical γ chains, also with 146 amino acids (4). At pH 6.8, when the adult hemoglobin binding curve is *e* in Figure 2.5, that of fetal hemoglobin F is close to curve *b*. The difference in behavior is attributable to DPG. As we shall see, DPG functions by binding to the β chains of adult hemoglobin A. It binds less well to the γ chains of hemoglobin F, which therefore can retain O_2 under conditions where adult hemoglobin has lost its oxygen. The overall oxygen transfer is a three-step process: from the lungs to the hemoglobin A of the mother, from there to the hemoglobin F of the fetus, and finally to the myoglobin of the fetal muscle to be stored until needed. After birth, hemoglobin F loses its special usefulness, and the synthesis of γ chains is gradually shut down. Within 4 to 6 months after birth the last fetal hemoglobin disappears and is replaced by the adult form.

Three other minor hemoglobin chains occur in man: δ, ε, and ζ. The first two resemble β and γ, and the third is α-like. Two early embryonic hemoglobins with chain compositions $\zeta_2\varepsilon_2$ (Gower-1) and $\alpha_2\varepsilon_2$ (Gower-2) disappear by the third month of pregnancy in favor of hemoglobin F; and hemoglobin A_2, with the composition $\alpha_2\delta_2$, is a minor (2.5%) constituent of adult blood. It is not clear what function hemoglobin A_2 has, or even whether it has any function different from that of hemoglobin A. There are some grounds for thinking that the δ chain is the product of a "failed" or a "spoiled" β-like gene. A higher ratio of δ to β chains is found in precursor cells in bone marrow on their way to becoming mature erythrocytes, and the decreased amount of δ in mature red blood cells could arise either because the δ gene is shut down before the β, or because the messenger RNA for the δ chain is unstable (6).

The foregoing has been a brief resumé of the physiological properties of hemoglobin that should be explainable in principle from a knowledge of the structure of the molecule: subunit cooperativity (all-or-nothing oxygen-binding behavior), and the sensitivity of O_2 binding to the presence of protons, carbon dioxide, chloride ions, and DPG. It is one of the triumphs of molecular biology that the behavior of hemoglobin *can* be explained at the molecular level, to an extent that is true for few other proteins. The first two protein crystal structure analyses were those of sperm whale metmyoglobin and horse methemoglobin (A1, A11), and these earned the Nobel Prize in chemistry for John C. Kendrew and Max F. Perutz in 1962. (The prefix *met-* signifies that the heme iron is in the oxidized Fe^{3+} state, rather than the reduced Fe^{2+} state as in the oxy and deoxy forms.) The met forms were experimentally the easiest to obtain, and the deoxy states also could be crystallized and studied with careful experimental techniques. The oxy forms proved more intractable: Unless extreme care is taken, O_2 oxidizes the heme iron from Fe^{2+} to Fe^{3+} rather than simply binding, thus yielding the unwanted met form of the molecule. As surrogates for oxy-hemoglobin and oxymyoglobin, structure analyses were carried out with other small molecules liganded (bound) to the heme irons in place of O_2: azide (N_3^-), cyanide (CN^-), fluoride (F^-), and carbon monoxide (CO). These are listed in Appendix 2.1. The most accurate, high-resolution structure analyses and refinements to date have been carried out for sperm whale met-, deoxy-, and oxymyoglobin (A4, A6, A7), horse methemoglobin (A13), and human deoxy- and carbonmonoxyhemoglobin (A18, A25). These are the basis for the highly detailed interpretation that now can be given of the way that the globin molecules work. (A detailed summary of myoglobin and hemoglobin structures is presented in an atlas by Fermi and Perutz [7].)

Figure 2.6 Four substances are physiologically important because they encourage oxyhemoglobin to drop its oxygens: protons, carbon dioxide, chloride ions, and 2,3-diphosphoglycerate (DPG). Each of these functions by binding more strongly to deoxyhemoglobin than to oxyhemoglobin, shifting the equilibrium to the right:

$$HbO_2 + X \rightleftarrows HbX + O_2$$

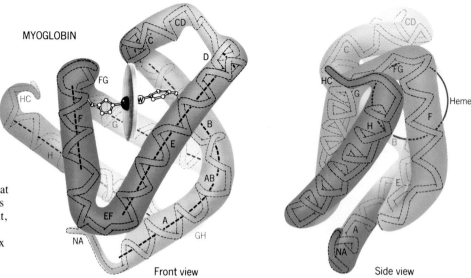

MYOGLOBIN

FG
CD
C
D
HC
F
W
G
B
H
E
AB
EF
A
NA
GH

Front view

CD
C
FG
HC
G
Heme
H
F
B
E
A
NA

Side view

Figure 2.7 The myoglobin molecule is built up from eight stretches of α helix that form a box for the heme group. Histidines interact with the heme to the left and right, and the oxygen molecule sits at point *W*. Helices E and F build the walls of the box for the heme; B, G, and H are the floor; and the CD corner closes the open end. The course of the main chain is outlined inside the colored cylinders.

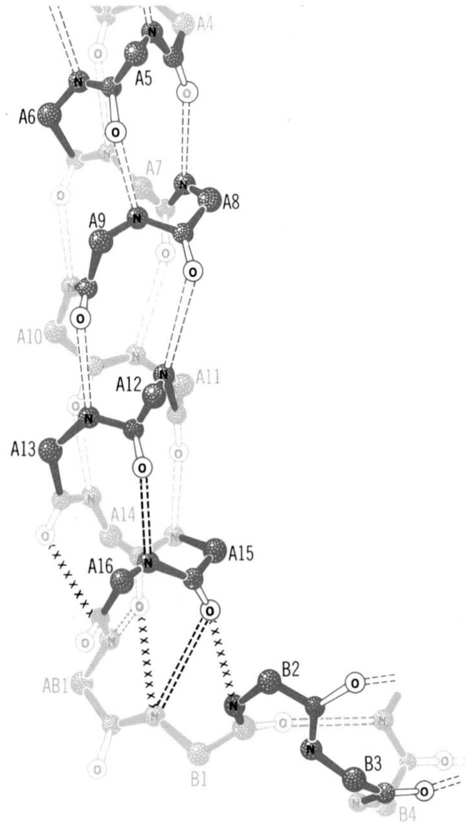

2.2 MYOGLOBIN, THE CONTAINER

The richest sources of myoglobin are the muscles of aquatic diving mammals such as seals, whales, and porpoises, which must store oxygen for relatively long periods. It was from sperm whale that Kendrew obtained myoglobin for the first x-ray structure analysis of a protein (A1–A9). The remarkable feature about the myoglobin molecule is that it is essentially a box for the heme group, built up from eight connected pieces of α helix. In Figure 2.7 these helices are shown as cylinders lettered A through H starting from the amino terminus. Interhelix bends are identified by double letters of the helices that they connect. All of the helices are right-handed, as are all the α helices ever observed in protein structures. If one begins to count helices at the first amino acid that contributes a C=O to a hydrogen bond with a residue farther down the chain, and ends at the last amino acid that contributes an H—N to a hydrogen bond with a residue earlier in the chain, then 131 residues are involved in helices and only 22 are not. The individual helices range in length from 4 amino acids (the first part of the F helix, termed the F′ helix) to 28 amino acids (the final H helix). These helices and the nonhelical regions that connect them are listed in Table 2.1 on page 31. As in Figure 1.12, an α helix has hydrogen bonds between the C=O of residue n and the H—N of residue $n + 4$. If the hydrogen-bond connection is one residue shorter, to the H—N of residue $n + 3$, then the helix is called a 3_{10} helix. If it is one residue longer, to $n + 5$, then it is called a π helix. All three of these helices are depicted in Figure 1.12. It is common in myoglobin for a stretch of α helix to be finished off by a tighter final turn of a 3_{10} helix (helices A, C, G, H), and less common to have a looser final turn as in a π helix (helix F).

A4
A5
A6
A7
A8
A9
A10
A11
A12
A13
A14
A15
A16
AB1
B2
B1
B3
B4

====== Actual hydrogen bonds

xxxxxx Hypothetical hydrogen bonds if the α helix were to continue beyond A16

Figure 2.8 Bending a corner between the A and B helices. The last α-helical hydrogen bond in the A helix is between the CO of residue A12 and the HN of residue A16. Thereafter the helix is tightened down and "pinched off" by two hydrogen bonds typical of 3_{10} helices: between the CO of A14 and the HN of AB1, and the CO of A15 and the HN of B1. Beyond B1 a new α helix begins, at right angles to the old one.

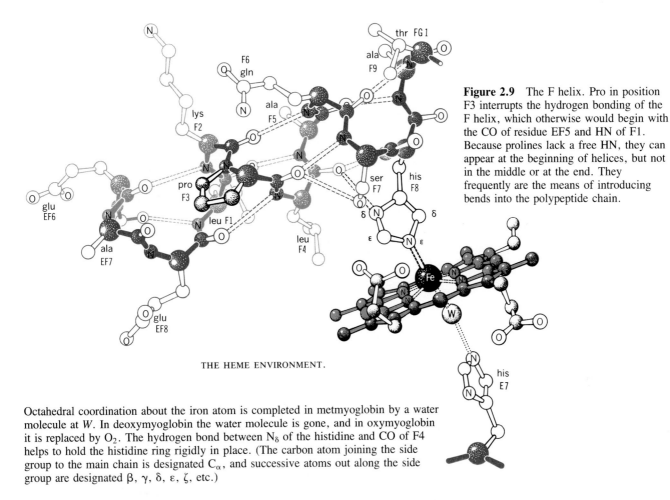

Figure 2.9 The F helix. Pro in position F3 interrupts the hydrogen bonding of the F helix, which otherwise would begin with the CO of residue EF5 and HN of F1. Because prolines lack a free HN, they can appear at the beginning of helices, but not in the middle or at the end. They frequently are the means of introducing bends into the polypeptide chain.

THE HEME ENVIRONMENT.

Octahedral coordination about the iron atom is completed in metmyoglobin by a water molecule at W. In deoxymyoglobin the water molecule is gone, and in oxymyoglobin it is replaced by O_2. The hydrogen bond between N_δ of the histidine and CO of F4 helps to hold the histidine ring rigidly in place. (The carbon atom joining the side group to the main chain is designated C_α, and successive atoms out along the side group are designated β, γ, δ, ε, ζ, etc.)

The myoglobin molecule as a whole is an oblate spheroid, approximately 44 by 44 by 25Å. The side view in Figure 2.7 shows how shallow the "box" really is. It is impossible to build up a globular molecule from α helices unless they are folded back on top of one another, so the polypeptide chain is forced to make sharp turns between these eight helices. Some of these turns are abrupt, with no nonhelical residues between, as from A to B, B to C, or D to E (Figure 2.8). If the angle between helix axes is smaller than a right angle, however, then a few intervening nonhelical residues are required to make the turn, as in the CD, EF, FG, and GH corners. The long E helix is bent slightly near its center without breaking any of its hydrogen bonds, and the F helix is broken into F′ and F segments by the presence of a proline residue in the middle (Figure 2.9). A proline is a sufficient but not a necessary requirement for a helix interruption and a bend in the chain; the sequences in Table 2.2 on page 32 show that the C and G helices begin with proline in myoglobin, and in both chains of hemoglobin also. The H helices also begin with proline in both chains of hemoglobin, but not in myoglobin. At these positions, prolines evidently are helpful but not essential.

The raison d'être of the myoglobin molecule is the heme group, to whose iron atom the oxygen molecule binds. The purpose of the heme and the polypeptide chain around it is to keep the ferrous iron from being oxidized (metmyoglobin, with a ferric iron, does not bind oxygen), and to provide a pocket into which the O_2 can fit. The eight helices are folded back and forth to construct a heme pocket with the E and F helices as sides, the B, G, and H helices for a floor, and the C, CD, and D region for a back wall (Figure 2.10).

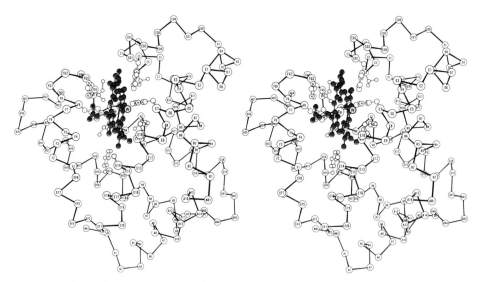

Figure 2.10 Stereo view of the main chain in myoglobin, with each amino acid represented by its labeled α carbon. A few key side chains near the heme are also shown: Thr C4, Phe CD1, His E7, Val E11, Ala E14, His F8, His FG3, Ile FG5, Leu G5, Ile G8, and Phe H15. For information on viewing glasses, see page 62.

The heme is completely surrounded by protein except for the edge that contains the two polar propionic acid side groups, which stick out of the pocket into the surrounding water. The hydrophilic or polar amino acids are spread uniformly over the surface of the molecule. Nearly every polar group on the surface is hydrogen bonded to a water molecule from the surroundings, so the protein is essentially coated with a layer of water one molecule deep. The strongly hydrophobic side chains (Val, Leu, Ile, Met, and Phe) appear on the inside of the molecule in two ways. Some of them line the inner surfaces of the α helices, where helices pack against one another. This undoubtedly helps the molecule to fold properly when its polypeptide chain is assembled at the ribosomes. Since an α helix has 3.6 residues per turn, the recurrence of hydrophobic side chains every three or four positions down the chain would favor folding into an α helix with one polar side and one hydrophobic or "oily" side, as is found in all the helices of myoglobin. The other hydrophobic residues in myoglobin form a lining for the heme pocket. The result of this folding-in of hydrophobic side chains is not a skeleton, as some of the earlier figures in this chapter might suggest. Rather, the molecule is a closely packed, compact object as in the space-filling computer-generated Figure 2.11a. But though this figure probably presents a better picture of what the myoglobin molecule would look like if we could see it in an imaginary x-ray microscope, skeletal drawings are better at showing the molecular anatomy.

Both ferric and ferrous iron normally prefer to be surrounded by six ligands in octahedral coordination. In myoglobin, four ligands are provided by the heme itself, and a fifth comes from His F8. The sixth position is the binding site for oxygen (Figure 2.9). In oxymyoglobin an O_2 molecule is present, with its O—O bond axis tilted 59° away from the normal to the heme plane (an Fe—O—O angle of 121°). In deoxymyoglobin this sixth site is vacant, and in metmyoglobin (with a ferric iron) a water molecule is at the O_2 site.

On the far side of the oxygen site lies the side chain of another histidine, His E7 (Figure 2.9). It is too far from the iron to complex directly with it, but its N_ε

MYOGLOBIN

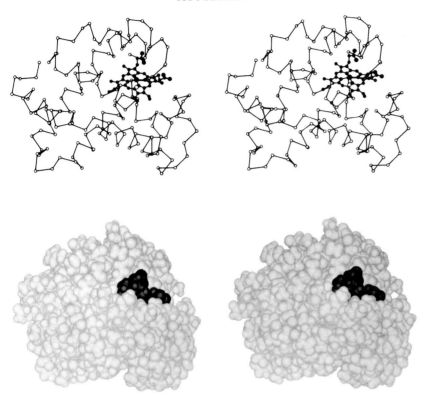

Figure 2.11 (a) Stereo pairs of sperm whale myoglobin. Top, ball-and-stick model showing only α-carbon atoms. Below, space-filling model with heme atoms darker, as in the top drawings. For information on three-dimensional models as an aid to visualizing myoglobin and hemoglobin, see page 62.

HEMOGLOBIN

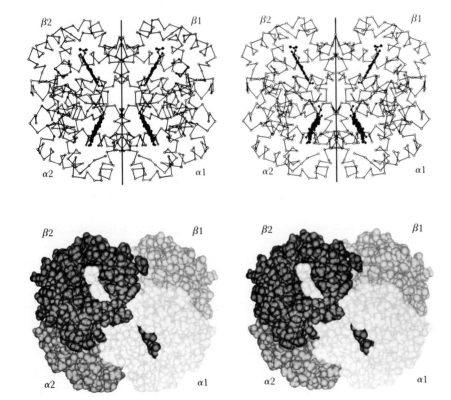

Figure 2.11 (b) The four chains of hemoglobin in stereo. This is the same view as in Figure 2.17a, which shows only the course of the main chain. Top, ball-and-stick model of α carbons. Heme atoms are black. Below, space-filling model of the surface. Hemes are shown in contrasting shades. (Stereos from Richard J. Feldmann, NIH. Reprinted by permission from *Biochemistry* by Wood, Wilson, Benbow, and Hood [2nd ed.], Benjamin/Cummings, Menlo Park, Calif., 1981.)

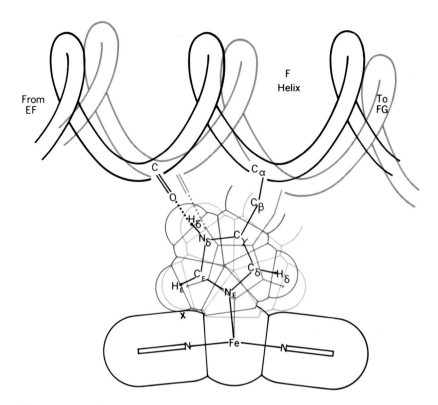

Figure 2.12 Interaction of His F8 and the F helix with the heme. In deoxymyoglobin (solid black and color), the iron atom is 0.55 Å out of the mean plane through all the atoms in the heme porphyrin, and the Fe—N_ε bond makes an angle of 11° with a perpendicular to the heme. In metmyoglobin (gray and light color), the iron atom is only 0.40 Å out of plane, and the Fe—N_ε is 4° away from the heme normal. The histidine can be regarded as essentially pivoting around its contact between H_ε and the heme, at x. Because His F8 is attached to the F helix through both its C_α—C_β bond and a hydrogen bond to a main-chain carbonyl group, the straightening up of the histidine forces the F helix toward the FG corner. (See Figure 2.29.) Outlines indicate approximate van der Waals boundaries of histidine atoms and heme rings.

makes contact with the oxygen or water molecule. Other small molecules and ions can also bind to myoglobin as the sixth iron ligand, including CO and NO to the ferrous form and NO_2^-, OH^-, F^-, CN^-, N_3^-, and H_2S to the ferric. Carbon monoxide, to our detriment, forms a particularly strong bond. Thirty to fifty times as much CO as O_2 will bind at equal concentrations of the two gases. For hemoglobin the situation is even worse: CO is favored over O_2 by a factor of 120 to 550, depending on conditions. In the presence of carbon monoxide, oxygen is displaced and the molecule is finished as an oxygen carrier. The victim smothers.

The heme group is not covalently bound to the globin (the polypeptide chain) other than by the histidine-to-iron coordination. The heme can be removed gently from the globin to form what is termed *apomyoglobin,* and then the original or a modified heme can be reinserted. The two heme propionates help to stabilize the heme by making hydrogen bonds to the side chains of His FG3 and Arg CD3. However, the main stabilizing forces for the heme appear to be hydrophobic contacts between the heme plane and the lining of the pocket. Several amino acid side chains are packed in van der Waals contact with the heme: Phe CD1, His E7, Thr E10, Val E11, Ala E14, Leu E15, Ser F7, His FG3, Ile FG5, Tyr G4, and Leu G5. Several of these are shown in Figure 2.10. Other side chains are packed against these to form three hydrophobic clusters to the left and right of the heme (as seen in the front view of Figure 2.7 or 2.10) and at the bottom of the heme pocket. But, strange as it may seem at first, none of these three clusters is tightly packed; each has some breathing room, or empty space. The empty space in the hydrophobic cluster at the right of the heme is the hole into which the O_2 molecule fits—but what purpose is served by the other two cavities? Crystallographers discovered that a xenon atom could be diffused into the hole in the cluster to the left of the heme, but this is hardly of any physiological significance. The answer, as we shall see when examining the different states of myoglobin (and, even more important, of hemoglobin), appears to be that the molecule requires a certain degree of flexibility in the vicinity of the heme group to allow a change from one conformation to another when oxygen binds, and to clear a space through which the oxygen molecule can enter and leave. If the heme were too densely packed amid protein side chains, no motion would be possible.

What differences are there between deoxymyoglobin and oxymyoglobin, other than the binding of the O_2 molecule? This has been a difficult question to answer, because it is not easy to bring O_2 next to the heme at room temperature without oxidizing the iron to produce metmyoglobin. However, high-resolution structure refinements of deoxymyoglobin (A6), metmyoglobin (A4), and oxymyoglobin at low temperature (A7), along with a neutron diffraction study of carbonmonoxymyoglobin (A8), have clarified the structural changes that are produced by oxygen binding. They are small but important, and become especially important in hemoglobin, where they are the key to heme–heme cooperativity.

The most obvious change is in the position of the iron atom relative to the heme plane (Figure 2.12). In deoxymyoglobin the iron has only five ligands: four from the heme itself, and the fifth from histidine. The iron is 0.55Å out of the mean heme plane toward the histidine, and the heme group itself is slightly domed in the direction of the histidine, with the four heme nitrogens 0.13 Å away from the best mean plane through all heme atoms. In metmyoglobin, the sixth position is occupied by a water molecule. Although H_2O is not a particularly strong binding ligand, it is strong enough to pull the iron atom 0.15 Å closer to the heme plane. (The doming of the heme is not changed.) The histidine pivots about its H_ε contact with the heme, making the bond between iron and the histidine nitrogen more nearly perpendicular to the heme plane than in deoxymyoglobin. In a linked motion, the F helix slides approximately 0.15 Å across the heme face in the direction of the FG corner (Figures 2.12 and 2.13). In oxymyoglobin and carbonmonoxymyoglobin, the motion that is observed in

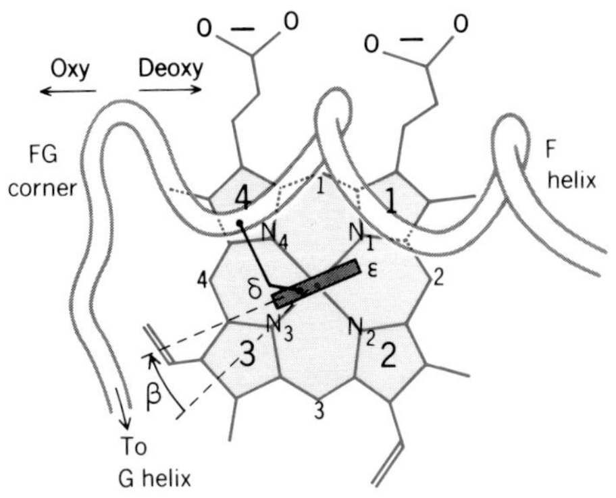

Figure 2.13 View of the heme region from the left in Figures 2.7 and 2.10, showing the way in which the F helix crosses the heme and is attached to it through His F8. In oxymyoglobin, as the histidine rocks forward on its H_ε atom and the iron atom moves farther into the heme plane, the F helix shifts 0.15 Å toward the FG corner (arrow pointing left). δ and ε indicate the two sides of the histidine as in Figure 2.12. The histidine plane is turned by an angle β away from the N_1–N_3 direction.

TABLE 2.1 HELICAL REGIONS IN MYOGLOBIN

| Nonhelical | Helical | Residues | Number of residues[a] | | Type and number of hydrogen bonds[b] |
			Nonhelical	Helical	
NA		1–2	2		
	A	3–20		17	α:12, 3_{10}:2
	B	20–36		17	α:13
	C	37–43		7	α:2, 3_{10}:1
CD		44–50	7		3_{10}:1
	D	51–58		7	α:4
	E	58–77		20	α:16
EF		78–81	4		
	F′	82–87		4	α:2
	F	86–96		11	α:7, π:2
FG		97–99	3		
	G	100–119		20	α:15, 3_{10}:1
GH		120–123	4		
	H	124–151		28	α:22, π:1, 3_{10}:1
HC		152–153	2		
			22	131	
		153			

[a]Counting the first residue to contribute a $C{=}O \cdots$ hydrogen bond, through the last residue to contribute a $\cdots H{-}N$. Residues that are shared between two helices are arbitrarily assigned to the second helix for counting purposes.

[b]3_{10}, α, and π indicate hydrogen bonds between the CO of residue n and the HN of residues $n + 3$, $n + 4$, and $n + 5$, respectively. See Chapter 1.

TABLE 2.2 SEQUENCES OF MYOGLOBIN AND HEMOGLOBIN CHAINS

The amino acid sequences of sperm whale myoglobin and the β and α chains of human and horse hemoglobin. Vertical bars of darker color indicate the same amino acid in all of the sequences shown here, while lighter bars apply only to hemoglobin.

MYOGLOBIN	NA1	—	NA2	A1	A2	A3	A4	A5	A6	A7	A8	A9	A10	A11	A12	A13	A14	A15	A16	AB1	B1	B2	B3	B4	B5	B6	B7	B8	B9	B10	B11
	1	—	2	3	4	5	6	7	8	9	10	11	12	13	14	15	16	17	18	19	20	21	22	23	24	25	26	27	28	29	30
	val	—	leu	ser	glu	gly	glu	trp	gln	leu	val	leu	his	val	trp	ala	lys	val	glu	ala	asp	val	ala	gly	his	gly	gln	asp	ile	leu	ile
HEMOGLOBIN β	NA1	NA2	NA3	A1	A2	A3	A4	A5	A6	A7	A8	A9	A10	A11	A12	A13	A14	A15	—	—	B1	B2	B3	B4	B5	B6	B7	B8	B9	B10	B11
	1	2	3	4	5	6	7	8	9	10	11	12	13	14	15	16	17	18	—	—	19	20	21	22	23	24	25	26	27	28	29
Human	val	his	leu	thr	pro	glu	glu	lys	ser	ala	val	thr	ala	leu	trp	gly	lys	val	—	—	asn	val	asp	glu	val	gly	gly	glu	ala	leu	gly
Horse	val	gln	leu	ser	gly	glu	glu	lys	ala	ala	val	leu	ala	leu	trp	asp	lys	val	—	—	asn	glu	glu	glu	val	gly	gly	glu	ala	leu	gly
α	NA1	—	NA2	A1	A2	A3	A4	A5	A6	A7	A8	A9	A10	A11	A12	A13	A14	A15	A16	AB1	B1	B2	B3	B4	B5	B6	B7	B8	B9	B10	B11
	1		2	3	4	5	6	7	8	9	10	11	12	13	14	15	16	17	18	19	20	21	22	23	24	25	26	27	28	29	30
Human	val	—	leu	ser	pro	ala	asp	lys	thr	asn	val	lys	ala	ala	trp	gly	lys	val	gly	ala	his	ala	gly	glu	tyr	gly	ala	glu	ala	leu	glu
Horse	val	—	leu	ser	ala	ala	asp	lys	thr	asn	val	lys	ala	ala	trp	ser	lys	val	gly	gly	his	ala	gly	glu	val	gly	ala	glu	ala	leu	glu

MYOGLOBIN	B12	B13	B14	B15	B16	C1	C2	C3	C4	C5	C6	C7	CD1	CD2	CD3	CD4	CD5	CD6	CD7	CD8	D1	D2	D3	D4	D5	D6	D7	E1	E2	E3	E4
	31	32	33	34	35	36	37	38	39	40	41	42	43	44	45	46	47	48	49	50	51	52	53	54	55	56	57	58	59	60	61
	arg	leu	phe	lys	ser	his	pro	glu	thr	leu	glu	lys	phe	asp	arg	phe	lys	his	leu	lys	thr	glu	ala	glu	met	lys	ala	ser	glu	asp	leu
HEMOGLOBIN β	B12	B13	B14	B15	B16	C1	C2	C3	C4	C5	C6	C7	CD1	CD2	CD3	CD4	CD5	CD6	CD7	CD8	D1	D2	D3	D4	D5	D6	D7	E1	E2	E3	E4
	30	31	32	33	34	35	36	37	38	39	40	41	42	43	44	45	46	47	48	49	50	51	52	53	54	55	56	57	58	59	60
Human	arg	leu	leu	val	val	tyr	pro	trp	thr	gln	arg	phe	phe	glu	ser	phe	gly	asp	leu	ser	thr	pro	asp	ala	val	met	gly	asn	pro	lys	val
Horse	arg	leu	leu	val	val	tyr	pro	trp	thr	gln	arg	phe	phe	asp	ser	phe	gly	asp	leu	ser	asn	pro	gly	ala	val	met	gly	asn	pro	lys	val
α	B12	B13	B14	B15	B16	C1	C2	C3	C4	C5	C6	C7	CD1	CD2	CD3	CD4	—	CD5	CD6	CD7	CD8	—	—	—	—	—	CD9	E1	E2	E3	E4
	31	32	33	34	35	36	37	38	39	40	41	42	43	44	45	46	—	47	48	49	50	—	—	—	—	—	51	52	53	54	55
Human	arg	met	phe	leu	ser	phe	pro	thr	thr	lys	thr	tyr	phe	pro	his	phe	—	asp	leu	ser	his	—	—	—	—	—	gly	ser	ala	gln	val
Horse	arg	met	phe	leu	gly	phe	pro	thr	thr	lys	thr	tyr	phe	pro	his	phe	—	asp	leu	ser	his	—	—	—	—	—	gly	ser	ala	gln	val

MYOGLOBIN	E5	E6	E7	E8	E9	E10	E11	E12	E13	E14	E15	E16	E17	E18	E19	E20	EF1	EF2	EF3	EF4	EF5	EF6	EF7	EF8	F1	F2	F3	F4	F5	F6	F7
	62	63	64	65	66	67	68	69	70	71	72	73	74	75	76	77	78	79	80	81	82	83	84	85	86	87	88	89	90	91	92
	lys	lys	his	gly	val	thr	val	leu	thr	ala	leu	gly	ala	ile	leu	lys	lys	lys	gly	his	his	glu	ala	glu	leu	lys	pro	leu	ala	gln	ser
HEMOGLOBIN β	E5	E6	E7	E8	E9	E10	E11	E12	E13	E14	E15	E16	E17	E18	E19	E20	EF1	EF2	EF3	EF4	EF5	EF6	EF7	EF8	F1	F2	F3	F4	F5	F6	F7
	61	62	63	64	65	66	67	68	69	70	71	72	73	74	75	76	77	78	79	80	81	82	83	84	85	86	87	88	89	90	91
Human	lys	ala	his	gly	lys	lys	val	leu	gly	ala	phe	ser	asp	gly	leu	ala	his	leu	asp	asn	leu	lys	gly	thr	phe	ala	thr	leu	ser	glu	leu
Horse	lys	ala	his	gly	lys	lys	val	leu	his	ser	phe	gly	glu	gly	val	his	his	leu	asp	asn	leu	lys	gly	thr	phe	ala	ala	leu	ser	glu	leu
α	E5	E6	E7	E8	E9	E10	E11	E12	E13	E14	E15	E16	E17	E18	E19	E20	EF1	EF2	EF3	EF4	EF5	EF6	EF7	EF8	F1	F2	F3	F4	F5	F6	F7
	56	57	58	59	60	61	62	63	64	65	66	67	68	69	70	71	72	73	74	75	76	77	78	79	80	81	82	83	84	85	86
Human	lys	gly	his	gly	lys	lys	val	ala	asp	ala	leu	thr	asn	ala	val	ala	his	val	asp	asp	met	pro	asn	ala	leu	ser	ala	leu	ser	asp	leu
Horse	lys	ala	his	gly	lys	lys	val	gly	asp	ala	leu	thr	leu	ala	val	gly	his	leu	asp	asp	leu	pro	gly	ala	leu	ser	asp	leu	ser	asn	leu

MYOGLOBIN	F8	F9	FG1*	FG2	FG3	FG4	FG5	G1	G2	G3	G4	G5	G6	G7	G8	G9	G10	G11	G12	G13	G14	G15	G16	G17	G18	G19	GH1	GH2	GH3	GH4	GH5
	93	94	95	96	97	98	99	100	101	102	103	104	105	106	107	108	109	110	111	112	113	114	115	116	117	118	119	120	121	122	123
	his	ala	thr	lys	his	lys	ile	pro	ile	lys	tyr	leu	glu	phe	ile	ser	glu	ala	ile	ile	his	val	leu	his	ser	arg	his	pro	gly	asp	phe
HEMOGLOBIN β	F8	F9	FG1	FG2	FG3	FG4	FG5	G1	G2	G3	G4	G5	G6	G7	G8	G9	G10	G11	G12	G13	G14	G15	G16	G17	G18	G19	GH1	GH2	GH3	GH4	GH5
	92	93	94	95	96	97	98	99	100	101	102	103	104	105	106	107	108	109	110	111	112	113	114	115	116	117	118	119	120	121	122
Human	his	cys	asp	lys	leu	his	val	asp	pro	glu	asn	phe	arg	leu	leu	gly	asn	val	leu	val	cys	val	leu	ala	his	his	phe	gly	lys	glu	phe
Horse	his	cys	asp	lys	leu	his	val	asp	pro	glu	asn	phe	arg	leu	leu	gly	asn	val	leu	ala	val	val	leu	ala	arg	his	phe	gly	lys	asp	phe
α	F8	F9	FG1	FG2	FG3	FG4	FG5	G1	G2	G3	G4	G5	G6	G7	G8	G9	G10	G11	G12	G13	G14	G15	G16	G17	G18	G19	GH1	GH2	GH3	GH4	GH5
	87	88	89	90	91	92	93	94	95	96	97	98	99	100	101	102	103	104	105	106	107	108	109	110	111	112	113	114	115	116	117
Human	his	ala	his	lys	leu	arg	val	asp	pro	val	asn	phe	lys	leu	leu	ser	his	cys	leu	leu	val	thr	leu	ala	ala	his	leu	pro	ala	glu	phe
Horse	his	ala	his	lys	leu	arg	val	asp	pro	val	asn	phe	lys	leu	leu	ser	his	cys	leu	leu	ser	thr	leu	ala	val	his	leu	pro	asn	asp	phe

MYOGLOBIN	H1	H2	H3	H4	H5	H6	H7	H8	H9	H10	H11	H12	H13	H14	H15	H16	H17	H18	H19	H20	H21	H22	H23	H24	H25	H26	HC1	HC2	HC3	HC4
	124	125	126	127	128	129	130	131	132	133	134	135	136	137	138	139	140	141	142	143	144	145	146	147	148	149	150	151	152	153
	gly	ala	asp	ala	gln	gly	ala	met	asn	lys	ala	leu	glu	leu	phe	arg	lys	asp	ile	ala	ala	lys	tyr	lys	glu	leu	gly	tyr	gln	gly
HEMOGLOBIN β	H1	H2	H3	H4	H5	H6	H7	H8	H9	H10	H11	H12	H13	H14	H15	H16	H17	H18	H19	H20	H21	HC1	HC2	HC3						
	123	124	125	126	127	128	129	130	131	132	133	134	135	136	137	138	139	140	141	142	143	144	145	146						
Human	thr	pro	pro	val	gln	ala	ala	tyr	gln	lys	val	val	ala	gly	val	ala	asn	ala	leu	ala	his	lys	tyr	his						
Horse	thr	pro	glu	leu	gln	ala	ser	tyr	gln	lys	val	val	ala	gly	val	ala	asn	ala	leu	ala	his	lys	tyr	his						
α	H1	H2	H3	H4	H5	H6	H7	H8	H9	H10	H11	H12	H13	H14	H15	H16	H17	H18	H19	H20	H21	HC1	HC2	HC3						
	118	119	120	121	122	123	124	125	126	127	128	129	130	131	132	133	134	135	136	137	138	139	140	141						
Human	thr	pro	ala	val	his	ala	ser	leu	asp	lys	phe	leu	ala	ser	val	ser	thr	val	leu	thr	ser	lys	tyr	arg						
Horse	thr	pro	ala	val	his	ala	ser	leu	asp	lys	phe	leu	ser	ser	val	ser	thr	val	leu	thr	ser	lys	tyr	arg						

*In the high resolution myoglobin refinement papers (A4, A6) FG1 through FG5 are designated as F10, FG1, . . . FG4, more accurately reflecting their true hydrogen bonding pattern. The older nomenclature has been retained in this table for uniformity with hemoglobin. Sequences from Reference 10 with minor corrections (48, A4, A6).

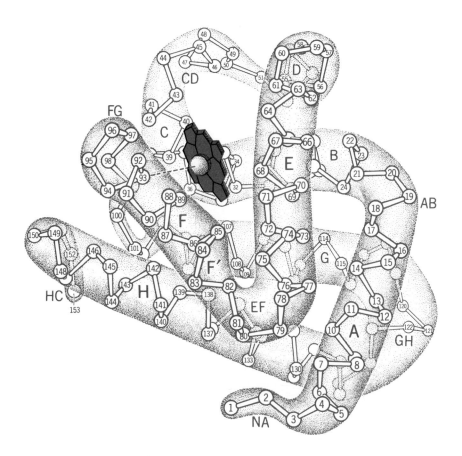

Figure 2.14 Deoxymyoglobin with sequential residues numbered from 1 to 153. Helix notation is in capital letters as in Table 2.2, opposite. The last half of the EF corner is now regarded as a turn of helix in its own right and is sometimes designated the F′ helix.

going from deoxy- to metmyoglobin is even more pronounced. The iron atom is only 0.26 Å out of the mean heme plane in the O_2 complex, and 0.24 Å out of plane in the CO complex, in rough agreement with the relative binding strength of H_2O, O_2, and CO to the heme iron. The shift in F-helix position in going from deoxy- to metmyoglobin pushes the FG corner away from the heme, and slightly compresses the 13 residues of the E helix nearest the EF corner. These changes are dissipated in the FG corner and E helix, and the rest of the molecule is essentially unchanged in deoxy and oxy states. These shifts are interesting and reasonable in myoglobin, but hardly of world-shaking significance. However, as we shall see, in hemoglobin they are the very foundation of heme–heme cooperativity.

To this point we have been identifying amino acid residues in myoglobin by their helix letter–number symbols. There are problems with these; they arose historically, and some residues that once were considered nonhelical are now included within α helices. Furthermore, minor differences in convention have arisen between myoglobin and hemoglobin terminology. Numbering the residues from 1 through 153 from the amino terminus is absolutely unambiguous, but then the parallelism of structure between myoglobin and each of the hemoglobin chains is obscured. Table 2.2, a "Rosetta stone" of globin notation, shows the amino acid sequences of sperm whale myoglobin and the α and β chains of horse and human hemoglobin. Both the sequential numbering and the helix notation are given for each chain. The sequential numbering is most nearly foolproof, as long as Table 2.2 is available to translate into helical and nonhelical regions. Figure 2.14 shows a standard drawing of sperm whale deoxymyoglobin with the residues numbered consecutively, and with the same helix notation as Figure 2.7.

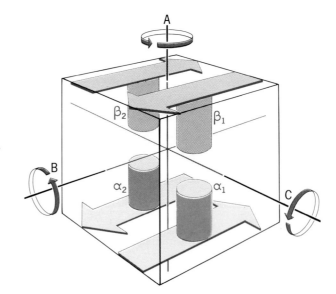

Figure 2.15 The symmetry of the hemoglobin molecule is shown by these four arbitrary asymmetric objects: α_1, α_2, β_1, and β_2.

Result of 180° rotation about:

A AXIS

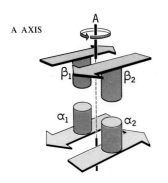

B AXIS

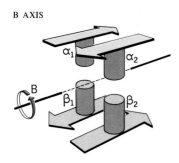

C AXIS

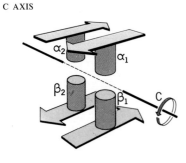

With two of type α and two of β, symmetry axis A is a true twofold axis, whereas B and C are both approximate or pseudoaxes of symmetry.

2.3   HEMOGLOBIN, THE CARRIER

Hemoglobin has been known for many years on chemical grounds to be made up of two α and two β chains. From the symmetry of the crystals, Perutz deduced as early as 1938 that the molecule consists of two identical halves related by a twofold axis (8)—that is, if one-half is rotated by 180° about a particular line, then it will superimpose on the other half. But it was not until 1960, when the first low-resolution x-ray structure analysis was completed (9), that it was realized that the α and β chains in one half molecule themselves are folded in a similar manner, and that both resemble myoglobin. The complete hemoglobin molecule nearly has what is termed *222 symmetry,* with three mutually perpendicular twofold axes intersecting at the center of the molecule.

The meaning of 222 symmetry is shown in Figure 2.15. The subunits shown in the figure—arrows attached to cylinders—bear no resemblance to the chains of hemoglobin, but their symmetry relationships are the same. If the entire assembly is given a 180° rotation about the vertical twofold axis marked A, then subunit α_1 superimposes on α_2, and β_1 superimposes on β_2.* Axis B would rotate subunit α_1 onto β_2, and α_2 onto β_1. But since the α and β subunits are only approximately the same, B is only a pseudosymmetry axis. Similarly, axis C is only a pseudoaxis of symmetry, since subunits α_1 and β_1 are not identical in hemoglobin, nor are α_2 and β_2.

One pathological type of hemoglobin with four β chains, hemoglobin H (also called β_4), does have molecules with ideal 222 symmetry since all four subunits are identical. This molecule is shown in Figure 2.16a, and in an exploded view in Figure 2.16b. Hemoglobin H is formed in a disease known as α-thalassemia, in which the patient produces fewer α chains or none at all. As a functional molecular machine, β_4 is a failure. It shows no cooperativity in oxygen binding, and has a hyperbolic binding curve (Figure 2.5) and high

---

*The subscripts to α and β merely identify relative positions in the molecule, and have no chemical significance. Unfortunately, subscripts are used both for this kind of identification, and also to designate the number of subunits in a tetramer, as $\alpha_2\beta_2$. These are both standard conventions, and there is no help for the potential confusion. You should be able to figure out which subunit convention is being used from context.

oxygen affinity like myoglobin. For reasons that we shall see shortly, the two different types of subunit, α and β, are necessary for the proper operation of the hemoglobin molecule. But hemoglobin H does illustrate a perfect symmetry with three perpendicular twofold axes, of a type that becomes only approximate in the $\alpha_2\beta_2$ hemoglobin A tetramer.

The actual arrangement of the two α and two β chains of horse methemoglobin is shown in Figure 2.17. The met form with its ferriheme was the first one whose structure was determined by x-ray diffraction. Although it closely resembles oxyhemoglobin, it is not identical to it. The molecule is roughly spherical, 64 by 55 by 50 Å. The four heme pockets, easily identifiable by their V-shaped E/F sides, are all exposed at the surface of the molecule. The heme groups of chains α_1 and β_2 are particularly close (Figure 2.17a), as are those of α_2 and β_1.

Each of the hemoglobin chains is folded in much the same way as a myoglobin molecule, with only minor differences. The *same* amino acid occurs in sperm whale myoglobin and in α and β chains of hemoglobin from man and horse at 26 positions along the chain. These are indicated by the darker color in Table 2.2, and are listed along with their function in Table 2.3. Most of these are hydrophobic side chains that pack against the heme or against one another in the interior of the molecule. Others are polar or charged side chains that form hydrogen bonds or salt bridges (ionic interactions) with other surface groups, and generally ensure that those regions of the chain will not fold into the interior of the molecule. His F8 and His E7 have unchanging roles as direct and indirect ligands to the heme iron. Positions B6 and E8 can only be glycines because they are the contact points where helices B and E cross, leaving no room for side chains between them. Other side chains in Table 2.3 interact with neighboring helices; of these, Tyr H23 will be seen to be involved in the hemoglobin mechanism. Pro C2 makes the sharp bend between B and C helices. Another proline performs the same role at the beginning of the G helix, but can be found at either position G1 or G2.

Figure 2.16 (a) The symmetrical but nonfunctional hemoglobin H (β_4) molecule is made up of four identical β chains, and occurs in a disease known as α-thalassemia in which too few or no α chains are produced. The molecule shows noncooperativity and high O_2 affinity, and in fact behaves like four myoglobin molecules that just happened to be connected. Because of the identity of all four subunits, however, the hemoglobin H molecule does show perfect 222 symmetry. (b) Exploded view of the hemoglobin H (β_4) subunits. This illustration shows more clearly how the four identical β subunits come together with 222 symmetry.

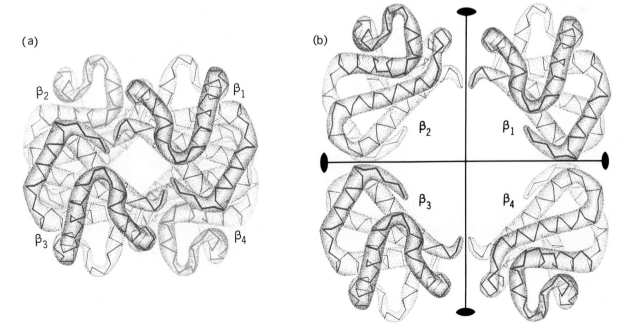

(a)

β_2 β_1

β_3 β_4

(b)

β_2 β_1

β_3 β_4

At 31 other positions along the chain, the same amino acid is found in horse and human α and β chains of hemoglobin, but a different residue is found in sperm whale myoglobin. These positions are marked by a light tint of color in Table 2.2. It is not as easy to explain why all these positions are invariant. Many are not invariant, of course, as soon as one looks at more hemoglobin sequences from different species. Many represent internal positions where a hydrophobic side chain is required, but the choice among valine, leucine, isoleucine, methionine, or even phenylalanine or tyrosine seems to be of little significance. Others are surface positions where one polar or charged side chain can be substituted for another of similar polarity. The positioning of hydrophobic and polar amino acids along the protein chain is one of the most important "codes" telling the protein how to fold properly in an aqueous environment.

HEMOGLOBIN TETRAMER

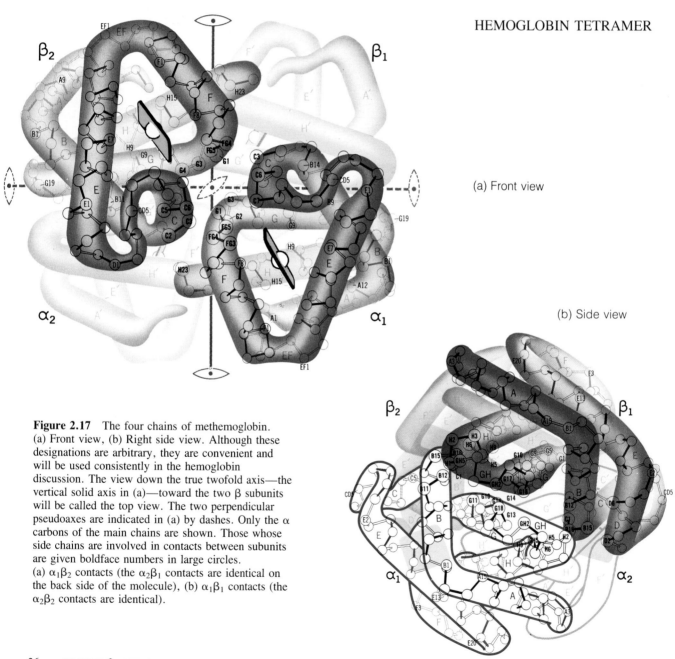

(a) Front view

(b) Side view

Figure 2.17 The four chains of methemoglobin. (a) Front view, (b) Right side view. Although these designations are arbitrary, they are convenient and will be used consistently in the hemoglobin discussion. The view down the true twofold axis—the vertical solid axis in (a)—toward the two β subunits will be called the top view. The two perpendicular pseudoaxes are indicated in (a) by dashes. Only the α carbons of the main chains are shown. Those whose side chains are involved in contacts between subunits are given boldface numbers in large circles. (a) $\alpha_1\beta_2$ contacts (the $\alpha_2\beta_1$ contacts are identical on the back side of the molecule), (b) $\alpha_1\beta_1$ contacts (the $\alpha_2\beta_2$ contacts are identical).

One significant difference between myoglobin and hemoglobin occurs at the intersubunit contacts of hemoglobin. Many of the side chains that are hydrophobic in hemoglobin must be polar in myoglobin because they are exposed to the polar surroundings. (This is more easily seen if we examine sequences from more species than the limited sample in Table 2.2. See Table 3.1 in the next chapter, or the more extensive tabulations in references 10–12.) Position B15, for example, is generally leucine or alanine in hemoglobin α chains, and valine, leucine, or isoleucine in β chains. In myoglobin it is the positively charged lysine. Position C1 is phenylalanine in α and tyrosine in β, but is histidine in myoglobin. C3 is usually threonine in α and always tryptophan in β, but glutamic acid in myoglobin. FG2 (myoglobin numbering) is leucine in both hemoglobin chains, but histidine in myoglobin. G17 is usually alanine in hemoglobin, but histidine in myoglobin. Other comparable examples can be found. The amino acid chosen at a particular position along a protein chain usually is remarkably well tailored for the role that the position has in that particular protein. This, of course, is because any amino acid sequence that we observe today is the result of a long, trial-and-error evolutionary selection process. We can learn much about the way in which a protein molecule operates, and its most essential and less critical regions, by looking at sequence com-

TABLE 2.3 AMINO ACID IDENTITIES IN MYOGLOBIN AND HEMOGLOBIN[a]

Amino Acid	Position	Function
Val	NA1	Beginning of chain
Leu	NA2	Contact with H helix
Val	A8	H helix contact; hydrophobic cluster at bottom of heme pocket
Trp	A12	Hydrogen bond to E helix
Lys	A14	External salt bridges
Val	A15	In hydrophobic cluster at bottom of heme pocket, as a spacer between B and G helices
Gly	B6	Close contact with Gly E8 where helices cross
Leu	B10	In hydrophobic cluster at right of heme
Arg	B12	In hemoglobin, hydrogen bond to Phe GH5 CO and to Gln H5 on neighboring subunit and salt bridge to Glu B8 of same subunit; in myoglobin, hydrogen bonds to water molecules
Pro	C2	Sharp turn between B and C helices
Thr	C4	Near heme
Phe	CD1	Packed against heme
Phe	CD4	In hydrophobic cluster at right of heme
Leu	CD7	In hydrophobic cluster at right of heme
Lys	E5	External salt bridges
His	E7	Interacts with sixth heme ligand
Gly	E8	Close contact with Gly B6 where helices cross
Val	E11	Packed against heme; in right hydrophobic cluster
Leu	F4	Packed against heme; in left hydrophobic cluster
His	F8	Fifth ligand to heme
Lys	FG2	Unknown
Leu	G16	Packed against A helix
Phe	GH5	In hydrophobic cluster at bottom of heme pocket, as a spacer between G and H helices
Lys	H10	External salt bridges
Lys	H22	External salt bridges
Tyr	H23	Hydrogen bond to C=O of Ile/Val FG5 to stabilize end of H helix

[a]Identical in sperm whale myoglobin and in horse and human α and β hemoglobin chains.

parisons of corresponding proteins from a great many species. This idea of molecular evolution will be developed in the next chapter.

The β chain of hemoglobin, with 146 residues, is shorter than the myoglobin chain (153 residues), mainly because its final H helix is shorter. The α chain shares this feature, and falls to only 141 residues because the D helix is also deleted. This can be seen in the sequences in Table 2.2, and in the side view of the hemoglobin structure in Figure 2.17b. The functional reason for the absence of the D helix in the α chains is not yet clear. It may have something to do with the proper positioning of the C helix and CD corner for the deoxy-to-oxy conformational change described later. Or it may have been only a random evolutionary accident that was accepted and propagated after it occurred, not because it was useful, but because it was harmless or neutral.

The packing of chains in the hemoglobin molecule is such that close, interlocking contact of side chains exists between unlike subunits, but there is little contact between α and α, or β and β. The αβ contacts are of two types. The $\alpha_1\beta_1$ or $\alpha_2\beta_2$ contacts involving B, G, and H helices and the GH corner (Figures 2.17b and 2.18) are called *packing contacts* because they represent subunit packing that is unchanged when the hemoglobin molecule goes from its deoxy to its oxy configuration. The $\alpha_1\beta_2$ or $\alpha_2\beta_1$ contacts involving mainly helices C and G and the FG corner (Figure 2.17a) are termed the *sliding contacts,* since they undergo the principal changes when there is a change in ligation state of the heme. As might be expected, the fixed packing contacts are more extensive than the variable sliding contacts: In deoxyhemoglobin, 126 atoms from 32 residues make up the packing contacts, and 107 atoms from 27 residues form the sliding contacts (A18). In methemoglobin, 35 side chains participate in packing contacts, and 18 participate in sliding contacts (A13). Approximately one-fifth of the total surface area of the isolated subunits is buried in the process of making the hemoglobin tetramer (13). Of this, 60% is involved in packing contacts and 35% in sliding contacts; the remaining 5% represents the small amount of contact between like subunits. These contacts are not merely hydrophobic. Hydrogen bonds and salt bridges also are important in holding the subunits together; approximately one-third of each of the contacts involves polar side chains.

2.4   SUBUNIT MOTION IN HEMOGLOBIN

The most obvious difference between deoxy- and oxyhemoglobin is that the subunits move relative to one another when a ligand such as O_2 binds to the hemes.* This motion is represented schematically in Figure 2.19. Each $\alpha_1\beta_1$ and $\alpha_2\beta_2$ half of the molecule moves as a rigid body, and the two halves slide over one another, rotating by 15° about a pivot passing through the α subunits. For this reason, the sliding-contact region between the FG corner of an α chain and the C helix of a β chain near the pivot point is termed the *flexible joint,* and that between the C helix of an α chain and the FG corner of a β chain farther away from the pivot is called the *switch region* (A25). The two α chains move very little relative to one another, aside from the 15° rotation, but the carboxyl ends of the H helices of the β chains come 7 Å closer together in oxyhemoglobin than in

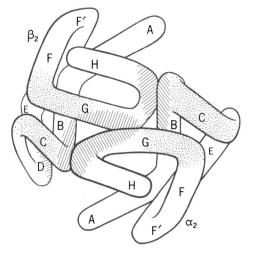

Figure 2.18   The $\alpha_2\beta_2$ dimer seen in a side view. Packing contacts (hatching) hold the dimer together. The action of the sliding contacts with the $\alpha_1\beta_1$ dimer (stipple) is demonstrated in Figure 2.19.

---

*Our information about the ligated states of hemoglobin has come from the refined structures of methemoglobin (A13) and carbonmonoxyhemoglobin (A25) as well as oxymyoglobin (A7). Since our interest is in oxyhemoglobin, however, the discussion will be expressed in terms of it, with the other ligated forms mentioned specifically only when it is suspected that they might differ from oxyhemoglobin.

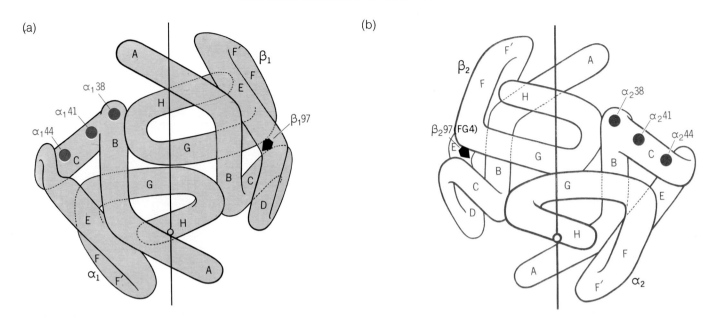

Figure 2.19 Subunit motion in hemoglobin. Side views of the separated $\alpha_1\beta_1$ and $\alpha_2\beta_2$ dimers, and their combination into deoxyhemoglobin and oxyhemoglobin. (a) The $\alpha_1\beta_1$ dimer (*gray*) is seen from outside the molecule, and the four critical residues appear on the undersides of the helices as seen here. (b) The $\alpha_2\beta_2$ dimer (color) is seen from inside the molecule. These two dimers are superimposed in (c) and (d). Critical α-chain residues in the switch region are in red. The critical $\beta97$ is in black.

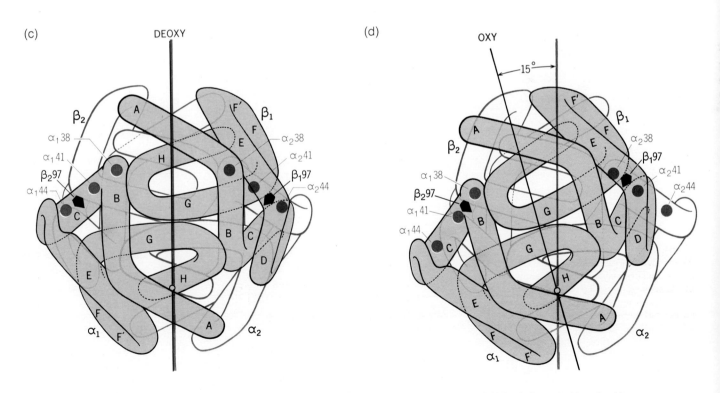

(c) The complete tetramer is shown in its deoxyhemoglobin conformation. Note the positions of $\beta97$ relative to $\alpha41$ and $\alpha44$.

(d) In oxyhemoglobin, the $\alpha_1\beta_1$ is rotated 15° relative to $\alpha_2\beta_2$. Note the new position of $\beta97$ between $\alpha41$ and $\alpha38$.

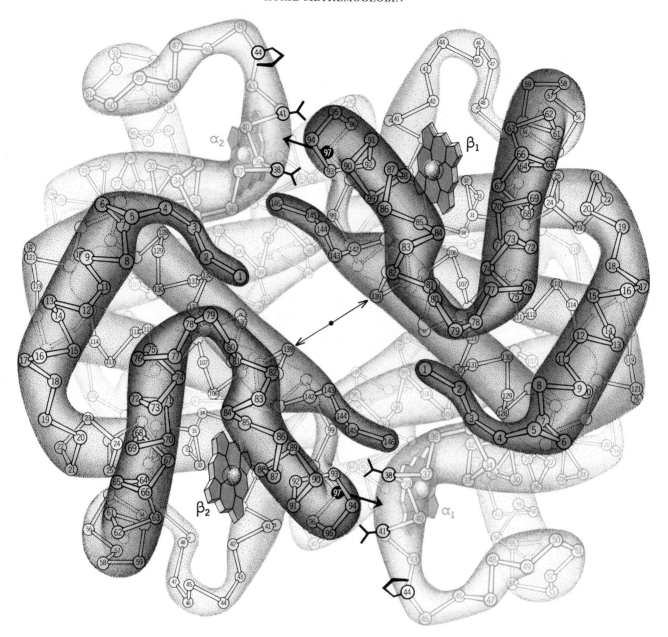

Figure 2.20 Top view of horse methemoglobin, with the subunit arrangement of oxyhemoglobin, showing the position of His β97(FG4) between Thr α38(C3) and Thr α41(C6). In the oxy-to-deoxy transformation, His β97 shifts to a new position, as shown in Figure 2.21 at the right. This shift of β chains changes the size of the DPG-binding site, as can be seen by comparing the different lengths of arrows across the central cavity. (Coordinates from Heidner, Ladner, and Perutz.)

deoxyhemoglobin. This shift in β subunit positions is easier to see in the top view, Figures 2.20 and 2.21. Now we can explain the effect of DPG that was mentioned earlier. DPG binds between the ends of the β chains in deoxyhemoglobin (Figure 2.23), where its negative charges can interact with the positive charges on the side chains of His 2(NA2), one of the two Lys 82(EF6), His 143(H21), and the amino termini of the β chains (Ref. A21). When the β chains come closer together in oxyhemoglobin, the DPG molecule is pushed out of its binding pocket. Conversely, by binding to the deoxy form, DPG shifts the equilibrium shown below to the right, favoring a release of oxygen:

$$Hb \cdot 4O_2 + DPG \rightleftarrows Hb \cdot DPG + 4O_2$$

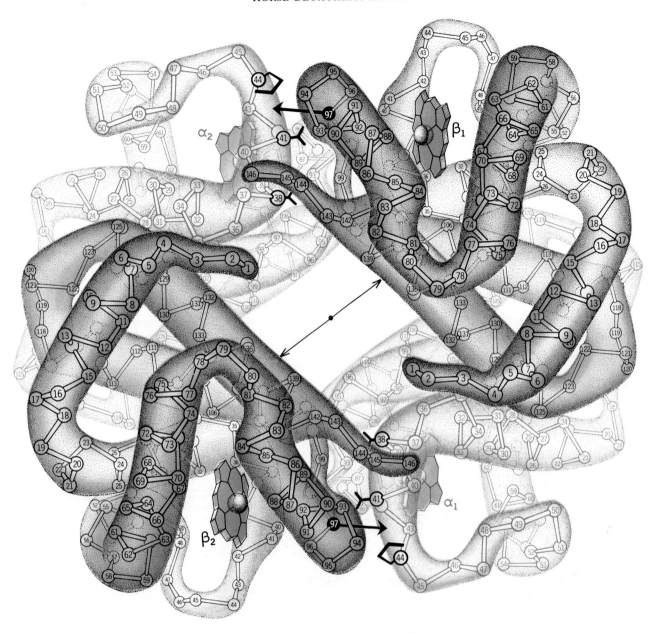

Figure 2.21 Top view of horse deoxyhemoglobin showing the shift of His β97 to its new position between Thr α41(C6) and Pro α44(CD2) as a result of the rotation of the $\alpha_1\beta_1$ dimer relative to $\alpha_2\beta_2$. Compare the top views on these two pages with the side views of Figure 2.19 to see how the relative rotation of dimers brings the β chains closer together in the oxy conformation and moves them farther apart in deoxy. (Coordinates from Perutz and Fermi.)

Inositol pentaphosphate (IPP), which performs the same O_2 regulatory role in birds that DPG does in mammals, binds even more strongly to the DPG site, as does inositol hexaphosphate (IHP).

The side-chain packing between the C helix of α subunits and the FG corner of β subunits in the switch region is different in deoxy- and oxyhemoglobin, as can be seen in Figures 2.20 and 2.21. In deoxyhemoglobin, His β97(FG4) nests between the side chains of Pro α44(CD2) and Thr α41(C6), whereas in oxyhemoglobin the histidine slips past the threonine and sits between it and Thr α38(C3). To this extent the oxy-to-deoxy transition is an either–or, two-state transition, and the term *switch* for this region is appropriate. But this is not to imply that other changes in the protein do not both precede and follow this particular change. The analogy of flipping a switch should not be taken too literally, other than as a convenient approximation. The slipping of the FG4 (β97) histidine between two positions along the opposing C helix can also be seen in Figure 2.19, where its relationship to the rotation of subunit pairs is more apparent.

More details of intersubunit side-chain contacts in deoxy- and oxyhemoglobin can be seen in Figure 2.22, in a front view looking directly into the $\alpha_1\beta_2$ sliding-contact zone, and these interactions are also listed in Table 2.4. In addition to the C–FG switch just mentioned, three other features of the contacts are notable: the packing of side chains in the flexible hinge region that remains the same in both states, a trade-off of hydrogen bonds between the two FG corners, and the network of bonds that tie down the carboxy termini of both α and β chains in deoxyhemoglobin. The side chains of residues 37 and 40 in the β subunit, and 42, 92, 94, and 95 in the α subunit, remain in contact in the joint region as the molecule goes from one conformation to the other. Farther up the diagram, a hydrogen bond between Asp β99(G1) and Asn α97(G4) in deoxyhemoglobin is replaced by one between Asp α94(G1) and Asn β102(G4) in oxyhemoglobin.

In deoxyhemoglobin, the carboxy termini of both the α and β chains are immobilized in a network of hydrogen bonds and salt linkages, all of which are broken in oxyhemoglobin. This, it turns out, is where much of the Bohr effect comes from. These bonds can be seen in Figure 2.22, but are clearer in Figure 2.24. The normal pK of an exposed histidine side chain is 6.5, and that of the free amino terminus of a protein is 8.0 (3). At the pH 7.4 of blood, the equilibrium expression

$$pH = pK + \log_{10}\frac{[X]}{[HX]}$$

TABLE 2.4 SUBUNIT CONTACTS IN HEMOGLOBIN AT THE $\alpha_1\beta_2$ INTERFACE

Contact region	Deoxyhemoglobin	Oxyhemoglobin
α_1FG/β_2C (flexible joint)	Arg $\beta_2$40(C6) against Arg $\alpha_1$92(FG4)	Same as deoxy
	Trp $\beta_2$37(C3) against Asp $\alpha_1$94(G1) and Pro $\alpha_1$95(G2)	Same as deoxy
α_1C/β_2FG (switch)	His $\beta_2$97(FG4) between Pro $\alpha_1$44(CD2) and Thr $\alpha_1$41(C6)	His between Thr $\alpha_1$41(C6) and Thr $\alpha_1$38(C3) instead
	H bond between Asp $\beta_2$99(G1) and Tyr $\alpha_1$42(C7)	H bond broken
FG corners	H bond between Asp $\beta_2$99(G1) and Asn $\alpha_1$97(G4)	H bond between Asn $\beta_2$102(G4) and Asp $\alpha_1$94(G1)
C helices	Arg $\beta_2$40(C6) against Tyr $\alpha_1$42(C7)	Same, plus H bond from Arg to CO of Thr $\alpha_1$41(C6)
Carboxy termini of α chains	Arg $\alpha_1$141(HC3) side chain H-bonded to Asp $\alpha_2$126(H9) side chain, and to CO of Val $\beta_2$34(B16). Salt-bridged through chloride ion to N terminus of opposite chain, Val $\alpha_2$1(NA1). Packed against Tyr $\beta_2$35(C1), Pro $\beta_2$36(C2), and Trp $\beta_2$37(C3)	Both Arg $\alpha_1$141(HC3) and Tyr $\alpha_1$140(HC2) freed to spend at least part of their time swung out in the surrounding solution. All bonds described for deoxy broken
	Arg $\alpha_1$141(HC3) C terminus salt-bridged to Lys $\alpha_2$127(H10) side chain	
	Tyr $\alpha_1$140(HC2) side chain H-bonded to CO of Val $\alpha_1$93(FG5). Ring tucked in $\alpha_2\beta_2$ interface, in contact with Pro $\beta_2$36(C2) and Trp $\beta_2$37(C3)	
	Tyr $\beta_2$35(C1) side chain H-bonded to Asp $\alpha_2$126(H9)	Same as deoxy, since α_2 and β_2 move as a unit
Carboxy termini of β chains	His $\beta_2$146(HC3) side chain H-bonded to Asp $\beta_2$94(FG1) side chain	Both His $\beta_2$146(HC3) and Tyr $\beta_2$145(HC2) freed to spend at least part of their time swung out into the solution. All bonds described for deoxy broken, including His β146$\cdots$Arg β94
	His $\beta_2$146(HC3) C terminus salt-bridged or H-bonded to Lys $\alpha_1$40(C5) side chain	
	Tyr $\beta_2$145(HC2) side chain H-bonded to CO of Val $\beta_2$98(FG5). Ring tucked in $\alpha_1\beta_1$ interface, in contact with Thr $\alpha_1$41(C6)	

See Figures 8 and 9 of Reference 7 for a more elaborate listing.

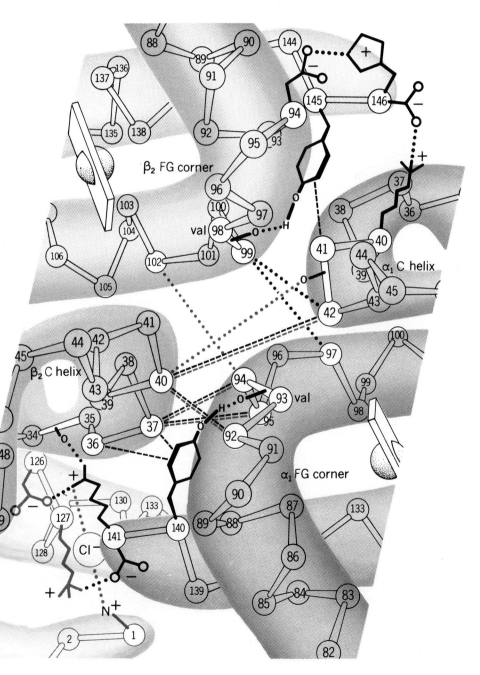

Figure 2.22 Front view of hemoglobin showing extensive subunit interactions between FG corners and C helices. The area outlined at left is enlarged below. Hydrogen bonds and salt bridges are shown as dotted lines, black for deoxyhemoglobin and colored for oxy. Nonbonded packing contacts are shown by black and colored dashed lines. Important interaction regions from top to bottom are the β-chain termini, switch region, flexible joint, and α-chain termini. Interactions are detailed in Table 2.4 at left. Red/green stereos from this same orientation are available for deoxy- and methemoglobin in diagrams D20 and D21 of Ref. 7.

Deoxyhemoglobin:

····· H bonds or salt bridges

----- Nonbonded packing contacts

Oxyhemoglobin:

····· H bonds or salt bridges

----- Nonbonded packing contacts

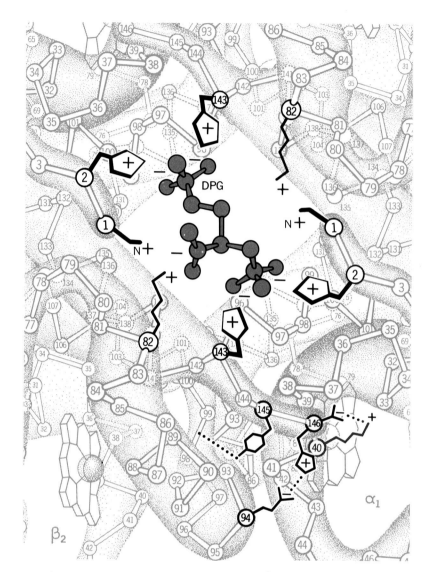

Figure 2.23 Amino acid side chains around the DPG-binding site. This top view of the central cavity in human deoxyhemoglobin shows the positive charges lining the DPG site: two each of the amino terminus, His β2(NA2), Lys β82(EF6) and His β143(H21). The DPG molecule with its five negative charges sits in the middle of this ring of positive charges. The fetal γ chain loses two of its eight positive charges by substituting Ser for His at β143, decreasing the affinity for DPG. Also shown are the salt bridges and the hydrogen-bonding pattern around the carboxyl terminus of the β chain (lower part of drawing), which emphasizes their contribution to the Bohr effect.

tells us that the ratio of unprotonated histidine [X] to the protonated form [HX] should be 8:1, or that only 11% of the histidines will be protonated. Similarly, the ratio of unprotonated or neutral amino termini [X] to the protonated form [HX] will be 1:4; only 20% of the amino termini will occur as —NH₂, with 80% as —NH₃⁺. But in deoxyhemoglobin, His β146 is stabilized in its positively charged form by the nearby negative charge of Asp β94, and a positive charge on the α amino terminus is similarly stabilized by the chloride ion that is bound between it and Arg α141. In these special environments, both groups essentially are completely protonated.

None of the bonds shown in Figure 2.24 occurs in oxyhemoglobin. At the β end of the molecule, Lys α40 moves out of range of the carboxy terminus of the β chain, and the hydrogen bond between Tyr β145 and the main-chain carbonyl group of Val β98 is weakened by a change in structure within the β subunit that will be described later. This is enough to break the salt link between His β146 and Asp β94, even though they are on the same subunit, and to release one Bohr proton. At the other end of the molecule, a combination of shifts in subunit structure (the H helices) and spacing between α subunits brings the carboxy termini 2 Å closer together than they were in deoxyhemoglobin. The Arg α141

DPG BINDING IN DEOXYHEMOGLOBIN

side chains are squeezed out, aided by a weakening of the Tyr α140 hydrogen bond as with the β chains, and the bonds shown in Figure 2.24a are broken. The chloride ions are lost, so the amino termini, lacking this charge stabilization, release more Bohr protons. In contrast, Arg α141 makes no contribution to the Bohr effect even though it occupies a position equivalent to His β146 at the other end of the molecule. Since the pK of arginine is 12.0, it is overwhelmingly protonated at pH 7.4 (99.997%), and remains effectively so whether the α carboxy terminus is bound or free.

The two His 146 on the β chains contribute 40% of the observed Bohr effect at pH 7.4 (14, 15); the two α termini contribute another 25%; yet another 10% comes from His α122(H5) (16). The reasons for the last contribution are unknown. Examination of this region in x-ray maps of deoxy-, met-, and carbonmonoxyhemoglobin shows no obvious changes that could account for the different degrees of protonation of the histidine (17). His β143(H21) and Lys β144(HC1), on the edge of the DPG-binding site (Figure 2.23), also are involved in the Bohr effect; in mutant human hemoglobin chains in which these are replaced by other amino acids, the Bohr effect is decreased. His β143 may possibly contribute a Bohr proton directly. However, replacing it by Gln or Pro, or replacing Lys β144 by Asn, also would upset the charge distribution around the DPG site and would loosen the carboxy terminal region of the β chains, setting free a Bohr proton from His β146.

The foregoing simple picture of the origin of the Bohr effect, attributing it mainly to His β146, the α amino termini, His α122, His β143, and Lys β144, is

Figure 2.24 Salt bridges and hydrogen bonds (the distinction is often unclear from x-ray analyses) between other groups and the last two residues in (a) the α chains and (b) the β chains of deoxyhemoglobin. All of these bonds are ruptured in oxyhemoglobin. As the β subunits move closer together, the bond between the β carboxy terminus and Lys α₁40(C5) is broken, allowing the end of the chain to swing free and leading to the breaking of interactions with Asp β₂94(FG1) and the CO of Val β₂98(FG5) also. At the other end of the molecule, a shift to the oxy configuration brings the α carboxy termini closer together also. The side chain of Arg α₁141(HC3) is squeezed out, rupturing all the bonds shown in (a). The two groups that contribute to the Bohr effect by becoming partially deprotonated in the oxy configuration are shown by colored plusses in circles.

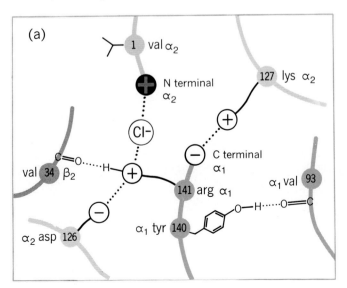

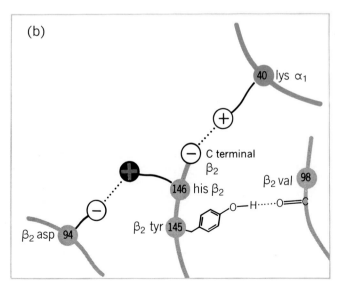

correct in general outline, but like any other understandable aspect of molecular biology, is to some extent a simplification. Ho and co-workers have found that His $\beta146$ contributes to the Bohr effect to a major extent under certain buffer conditions, but less so under others that they consider closer to physiological conditions (18). Gurd has also carried out energy calculations that suggest that as many as 11 different histidines could contribute to the Bohr effect, in some cases in association with bound chloride ions like that at the α termini (19). The Perutz–Kilmartin model presented in the previous paragraphs should be considered as a first-order approximation, but the full Bohr effect is probably the result of many small contributions from many side chains whose environment is altered during the T-to-R subunit transition.

The reasons why DPG, H^+, and Cl^- all promote the release of O_2 now are clear. DPG binds between the β chains of deoxyhemoglobin, but is ejected from the oxy form. H^+ protonates His $\beta146$, the amino termini of the α chains, and perhaps His $\alpha122$ and His $\beta143$, to a greater extent in deoxyhemoglobin than in oxy. Chloride ions assist protonation of the α amino termini in deoxyhemoglobin, but do not bind to oxyhemoglobin because the network of positive charges shown in Figure 2.24a is broken up and dispersed. All three— DPG, H^+, and Cl^-—act as effectors, X, shifting the following equilibrium to the right:

$$Hb \cdot 4O_2 + nX \rightleftharpoons Hb \cdot nX + 4O_2$$

The number of effectors, n, per tetrameric hemoglobin molecule is 1 for DPG and about 2 for chloride ions and protons (A14).

Chloride ions also help to lower the oxygen affinity of hemoglobin in another way that at first may appear paradoxical. They and other anions can decrease O_2 affinity in the absence of DPG, by binding within the ring of positive charges at the DPG site. In fact, any change that decreases the net positive charge within this site diminishes O_2 binding. There is decreased affinity for O_2 in human mutant hemoglobins in which Lys $\beta82$ is replaced by Met, Asn, or Asp, or Gly $\beta134$ is replaced by Asp. Conversely, an increase of net positive charge at this site enhances O_2 binding. Mutants in which His $\beta2$ or $\beta143$ becomes Arg, Asp $\beta79$ becomes Gly, or Asn $\beta80$ becomes Lys, all show increased O_2 binding (20). The apparent paradox arises when one examines Figures 2.20 and 2.21 and sees that these groups ringing the DPG site are *closer together* in the oxy- hemoglobin configuration than in deoxy. Shouldn't elimination of positive charges then favor the oxy state more than deoxy, leading to increased O_2 affinity? The resolution of the paradox comes when one realizes that the charge effect operates, not on the oxy-to-deoxy subunit equilibrium, but on the de- oxyhemoglobin subunits themselves. Anions can produce a similar decrease in oxygen affinity in isolated β or γ chain subunits (21). The reason for this is not yet known, but it is a separate phenomenon from the preferential locking into the deoxy state that DPG produces when it slips into the opening between the ends of the β subunits. DPG binds where it does in part because of the positive charges surrounding the cavity, but the neutralization of these positive charges is not the mechanism by which the lowered O_2 affinity is produced. That follows from the shift in equilibrium to the right produced because DPG cannot bind in a comparable manner to the oxyhemoglobin molecule:

$$Oxyhemoglobin + DPG \rightleftharpoons deoxyhemoglobin \cdot DPG$$

What is the structural basis for weaker DPG binding in the γ chain of fetal hemoglobin, in comparison with the β chain of the normal adult form? Weaker DPG binding means that fetal hemoglobin can maintain a higher affinity for O_2 in the presence of DPG, facilitating the transfer of O_2 from the blood of the mother to that of the fetus. The sequences of both human and chimpanzee γ chains have two suggestive differences: an uncharged Ser at position β143 in place of the His, Lys, or Arg always found in β and δ chains, decreasing the attraction for DPG, and a bulky Phe in place of Leu at postion β3. The latter substitution may displace the amino terminus from its normal position, removing both the terminal NH_3^+ and the His β2 side chain from the DPG site. With as many as six of the eight positive charges displaced, the site may no longer bind DPG effectively.

How does carbon dioxide favor deoxygenation? It carbamylates the neutral (uncharged) amino termini of the α subunits in oxyhemoglobin, converting them to anions that can interact directly with Arg α141 even without chloride ions, hence favoring a shift to the deoxy configuration:

$$-NH_3^+ \underset{\substack{\text{normal} \\ \text{protonation} \\ \text{equilibrium}}}{\rightleftharpoons} -NH_2 + H^+ \xrightarrow[\substack{\text{carbamylation} \\ \text{reaction}}]{+CO_2} -NH-COO^- + 2H^+$$

This reaction releases protons, which also favor the deoxy form by combining with His β146. The amino termini of the β chains can be carbamylated as well, but here the release of protons that favors deoxyhemoglobin is balanced by a disruption of DPG binding by introducing two negative charges into the binding site, hence favoring the oxyhemoglobin conformation. This binding of as many as four carbon dioxide molecules per hemoglobin tetramer is a direct way for hemoglobin to transport carbon dioxide back to the lungs after it has dropped its oxygen. The soaking up of protons that result from the bicarbonate reaction,

$$H_2O + CO_2 \rightarrow HCO_3^- + H^+$$

provides an indirect means of hemoglobin-assisted CO_2 transport.

2.5   THE ALLOSTERIC MODEL

The Bohr effect and the influence of effectors have been accounted for structurally, but nothing has been said yet to explain heme–heme cooperativity and the sigmoid oxygen-binding curve for hemoglobin seen in Figure 2.5. In 1965, Monod, Wyman, and Changeux proposed their theory of *allostery* ("different shape") to explain feedback control in enzymes (22). In this theory, the activity of an enzyme toward its substrate can be modified by the binding of molecules (the effectors) that need have no structural resemblance to the true substrate, and need not bind anywhere close to the enzymatic active site. This clearly is different from competitive inhibition at the active site by inhibitors that resemble the proper substrate. It offers the possibility that an enzyme that catalyzes an early reaction in a metabolic pathway can be shut down by an excess of product molecules much farther down the pathway, an obviously efficient kind of feedback control. The model assumes a multisubunit enzyme that can exist in only two different conformations: a T or "tense" state with low or zero affinity for substrate, and an R or "relaxed" state with high affinity for substrate. The microscopic association constants for interaction of substrate with subunits in the T and R states are A_T and A_R, and their ratio, A_T/A_R, is denoted by c. This ratio,

c, is assumed to be quite small, since the substrate binds more tightly to R than to T. (The ratio would be zero if the T state had no substrate affinity.) A change of state of the molecule involves simultaneous change in all subunits. If there are only two subunits, for example, then T = tt or R = rr configurations are permitted, but the mixed configuration tr is not. In the absence of substrate, T and R molecules are in equilibrium,

$$T_0 \rightleftharpoons R_0$$

and the equilibrium constant is

$$L = \frac{[T_0]}{[R_0]}$$

L is assumed to be very large, since in the absence of substrate most molecules will be in the T state. The T-to-R equilibrium shown is a dynamic one, of course, but when a substrate molecule binds to one of the subunits of an enzyme in the R state, it tends to lock the entire molecule in the R conformation, making the other subunits easy targets for more substrate. This is the basis for subunit "cooperativity," whereby the binding of later substrate molecules is made easier by the binding of the first one. This equilibrium allosteric model even works in extreme cases where $c = 0$ and the T state has *no* affinity for substrate.

If another unrelated molecule binds preferentially to either the T or the R conformation of a subunit, then it can act as an *allosteric effector,* modifying the behavior of the enzyme. If it binds better to the T state, then it diminishes substrate binding and is called an *allosteric inhibitor,* with negative feedback control or damping. If it favors the R state, then it is an *allosteric activator,* with positive feedback control or amplification. Examples of both are known in biological reactions.

Although hemoglobin is not an enzyme, it can be regarded as an allosteric molecule in which the substrate is O_2 and the reaction is one of simple binding rather than binding followed by catalysis. Deoxyhemoglobin then is the T state with low (but not zero) O_2 affinity, and oxyhemoglobin is the R state with high affinity. Protons, chloride ions, and DPG all are allosteric inhibitors, decreasing the binding of oxygen although they neither resemble the oxygen molecule nor bind at the same place. The experimental data on oxygen binding to adult human hemoglobin at pH 7.4 are well fitted by a ratio of association constants, c, around 0.003 to 0.03, and $L = 10^4$ (23, 24). Adding one DPG molecule per hemoglobin tetramer shifts the equilibrium in favor of the T state, with an increase of L to 10^6; the same amount of IHP raises L to 10^8. Lowering the pH by 1 unit (increasing the H^+ concentration by a factor of 10) has about the same effect on L as adding an equimolar quantity of DPG.

For the tetrameric hemoglobin molecule, let T_n be the deoxy subunit configuration with n oxygen molecules bound to its hemes, and let R_n be a molecule in the oxy subunit configuration with the same number of oxygens. Although so far we have considered only the extreme states, T_0 and R_4, one can set up a general equilibrium between subunit conformation and extent of oxygenation:

$$
\begin{array}{ccccccccc}
T_0 & \underset{-O_2}{\overset{+O_2}{\rightleftarrows}} & T_1 & \underset{-O_2}{\overset{+O_2}{\rightleftarrows}} & T_2 & \underset{-O_2}{\overset{+O_2}{\rightleftarrows}} & T_3 & \underset{-O_2}{\overset{+O_2}{\rightleftarrows}} & T_4 \\[4pt]
\updownarrow L & & \updownarrow Lc & & \updownarrow Lc^2 & & \updownarrow Lc^3 & & \updownarrow Lc^4 \\[4pt]
R_0 & \underset{-O_2}{\overset{+O_2}{\rightleftarrows}} & R_1 & \underset{-O_2}{\overset{+O_2}{\rightleftarrows}} & R_2 & \underset{-O_2}{\overset{+O_2}{\rightleftarrows}} & R_3 & \underset{-O_2}{\overset{+O_2}{\rightleftarrows}} & R_4
\end{array}
$$

If the equilibrium constant for the conformation change with no ligand present is

$$\frac{[T_0]}{[R_0]} = L$$

then that for molecules with one ligand bound is

$$\frac{[T_1]}{[R_1]} = \frac{[O_2][T_0]A_T}{[O_2][R_0]A_R} = Lc$$

and those for the successive steps are Lc^2, Lc^3, and Lc^4, as shown above. If we use $L = 10^4$ and $c = 0.01$, then the ratio of unliganded T_0 to R_0 is 10,000 to 1, T_2 and R_2 are present in equal concentrations, and the ratio of T_4 to R_4 is 1 to 10,000. Hence we probably could have neglected R_0 and T_4 entirely, but they are included here for completeness.

When the first O_2 binds to a T-configuration molecule, a certain amount of strain is introduced. (We will see the molecular basis for this strain shortly.) This strain could be reduced if the molecule were to relax to the R state, and in fact is responsible for the difference in association constants A_T and A_R. Successive addition of more O_2 molecules to the T-state molecule increases the total strain, until finally the transition from T to R occurs. All of the subunits then have a higher affinity for O_2, so the last subunits bind O_2 more easily. For hemoglobin under physiological conditions, the transition from T to R can be thought of as occurring on the average after two or three O_2 have bound (25). Conversely, when a fully oxygenated R_4 molecule loses one or two of its oxygens, it switches back into the low-affinity T state and drops the last oxygens more easily. This is consistent with the behavior of hemoglobin, and leads to sigmoid heme–heme interaction curves that fit the observed data—but what is the *structural* basis for such an allosteric transition in hemoglobin? What is the "trigger" that produces a T-to-R molecular subunit transition after two or three O_2 have bound?

2.6   CHANGES WITHIN SUBUNITS

Prior to the high resolution structure refinements of myoglobin and hemoglobin, it had been proposed that the size of the iron atom might be the decisive factor in triggering the subunit transition. Model x-ray studies with porphyrin compounds had shown that a five-coordinated high-spin Fe(II) iron sits roughly 0.45 Å out of the heme plane, whereas a sixth coordinating ligand pulls the now low-spin iron into the plane (A15). Hence the binding of O_2 to hemoglobin would force the iron atom into the heme plane, pushing the heme closer to His F8 and the F helix, and this motion could be propagated into an eventual T-to-R (deoxy-to-oxy) subunit transition. The problem was that the details of this propagation process were neither clear nor very convincing.

The high-resolution refinements have provided a plausible answer, which is consistent with NMR and spectroscopic evidence, and with theoretical energy calculations. The key is an exaggerated version of the tertiary structure change within each subunit that we have already seen in myoglobin (Figure 2.25 and Table 2.5). In both deoxymyoglobin and deoxyhemoglobin, the histidine bond to the iron atom is tilted away from a perpendicular to the heme plane (11° for myoglobin and 7° or 8° for hemoglobin—probably identical within the limits of error of the structure analyses). The iron atom lies 0.6 Å out of the mean plane of

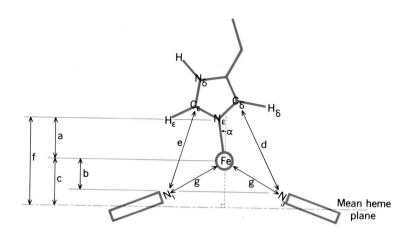

Figure 2.25 Geometry of His F8, iron, and the heme in deoxy and liganded globins. For values of the indicated parameters from high-resolution x-ray structure refinements, see Table 2.5. In the most highly refined structures, the heme has been found to be domed slightly toward His F8, with the four heme nitrogens closer to the iron, *b*, than the average heme atom plane, *c*.

the porphyrin nitrogens and carbons. In contrast, in all of the various liganded forms—met (with H_2O), carbonmonoxy, or oxy—the histidine–iron bond is more nearly perpendicular and the iron atom is closer to the heme plane. This out-of-planeness of the iron atom in the deoxy state owes more to a pyramidal doming of the porphyrin skeleton of the heme than to simple extraction of the iron from a rigidly planar heme. EXAFS (extended x-ray absorption fine structure) spectroscopic measurements show that the distance between iron and the four nitrogens in the porphyrin ring (*g* in Figure 2.25) changes very little—2.055 ± 0.01 Å in deoxyhemoglobin versus 1.98 ± 0.01 Å in oxyhemoglobin (26)—and the most highly refined x-ray analyses agree.

The asymmetric tilt of His F8 in the deoxy state, and its straightening up in oxy, are also detectable by comparing the distances between the δ and ε carbon atoms in the histidine ring and their closest heme nitrogens (distances *d* and *e* in Figure 2.25). In carbonmonoxyhemoglobin the two are the same within 0.1 Å; in deoxyhemoglobin, however, *d* is longer than *e* by 0.6–0.7 Å. (The numbers for myoglobin are not directly comparable because the histidine ring moves laterally slightly as well as tilting.) To a first approximation one can regard the shift as a rocking of histidine about the nonbonded contact between its ε hydrogen atom and the heme plane (Figure 2.12), but this is not strictly accurate, since the histidine also moves 0.2–0.5 Å closer to the heme in the six-coordinated state. (Compare distance *e* in deoxyhemoglobin and carbonmonoxyhemoglobin in Table 2.5.)

An out-of-plane iron atom in a domed porphyrin ring is in an unfavorable position for binding a sixth ligand on the opposite side of the heme plane. For the sixth ligand to be added easily, His F8 must straighten up and move closer to the heme. It is restrained from doing so in the deoxy or T configuration by several factors, of which the old explanation of a large iron radius now seems to be the least important. The histidine cannot simply sink far enough toward the heme plane because of steric hindrance between its ε hydrogen and the heme. It cannot freely straighten up its 8° tilt because of its attachment to the F helix and the packing of other side chains around it. As with myoglobin, although the histidine ring is not so tightly packed that it cannot move, the packing is close enough that an 8° reorientation would require adjustments and propagation of the disturbance through neighboring side chains. Figure 2.26 shows the approximate van der Waals nonbonded packing outlines of His F8 and its immediate neighbors, viewed from the F-helix side in the same orientation as that of Figure 2.13. Val FG5 is packed against the vinyl side chain of ring 3 of the heme, which will turn out to be important in passing information about the ligation state of one heme on to the rest of the molecule.

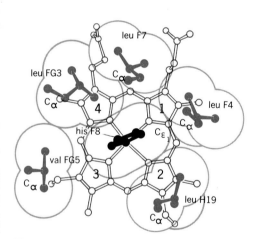

Figure 2.26 Packing of side chains on the His F8 side of the heme in the β subunit of hemoglobin. The view is identical to that of the myoglobin heme in Figure 2.13, and the α hemoglobin subunit in Figure 2.27. The histidine is surrounded by a cage of hydrophobic side chains. Val FG5 is packed against the vinyl group of ring 3 of the heme, and is pushed away when the heme moves following ligand binding. (Adapted from reference 24.)

TABLE 2.5 HEME GEOMETRY IN GLOBINS[a] *See Figure 2.25*

	Deoxy			Met			Oxy	Carbonmonoxy		
	Mb	Hb α	Hb β	Mb	Hb α	Hb β	Mb	Mb	Hb α	Hb β
His plane orientation (β in Figure 2.13)	19°	20°	25°	19°	21°	15°	6°	19°	14.5°	11.5°
α = angle between Fe—N$_\varepsilon$ bond and heme normal	10.7°	8°	7°	3.9°	5°	5°	4°	—	0.9°	1.1°
DISTANCES IN (Å)										
a = Fe—N$_\varepsilon$	2.0	2.0(30)	2.2(30)	2.13	2.1	2.2	2.1	—	2.09	2.08
b = Fe to heme N plane	0.42	b	b	0.27	b	b	0.16	0.10(10)	0.00	−0.02
c = Fe to heme mean plane	0.52	0.6(20)	0.63(20)	0.40	0.07(06)	0.21(06)	0.19(03)	0.24	0.03(20)	0.00(20)
f = N$_\varepsilon$ to heme mean plane	2.6	2.6(30)	2.8(30)	2.52	2.2	2.4	2.3	2.4	2.12	2.09
g = Fe to heme N atoms (avg)[c]	2.06	2.1(10)	2.1(10)	2.04	—	—	1.95(06)	2.02	2.00	2.00
d = C$_\delta$ to N$_3$ distance	3.5	3.8(30)	4.2(30)	3.4	—	—	—	—	3.10(26)	3.06(26)
e = C$_\varepsilon$ to N$_1$ distance	3.4	3.2(30)	3.5(30)	3.3	—	—	—	—	3.00(26)	2.99(26)
rms errors in atomic positions	0.28	0.40		0.31	0.25		—	—	0.55	
Reference	A5[d]	A18, A5[d], 46		A4[d]	A13		A7	A8[d]	A25[d]	

[a]Values in parentheses are probable errors in hundredths of an angstrom (e.g., 2.09(10) = 2.09 ± 0.10).
[b]Effectively the same as c, since the heme was assumed to be flat during refinement.
[c]EXAFS spectroscopy yields 2.055 ± 0.01 Å for the iron-to-heme nitrogen distance in deoxyhemoglobin and 1.98 ± 0.01 Å in oxyhemoglobin, in excellent agreement with these x-ray results (23, 46).
[d]And personal communication.

The actual shifts that are observed in the α subunit when one compares deoxyhemoglobin with carbonmonoxyhemoglobin (A25) appear in Figure 2.27. The F helix moves 1.4 Å to the left along its axis, shifts 0.7 Å downward in the figure, and sinks 0.4 Å closer to the heme. The heme shifts 0.5 Å to the left and 0.4 Å farther into the heme pocket, but does not tilt or move perpendicular to the plane of the diagram. The net result is that the F helix slides 1.0 Å to the left across the face of the heme. These disturbances are propagated back along the E and G helices, but are damped down halfway along them, as Figure 2.27 shows, leaving the remainder of the α subunit essentially unchanged.

Changes in the β subunit in going from deoxy- to oxyhemoglobin are similar: Its F helix moves 0.9 Å to the left in the orientation of Figure 2.27, shifts

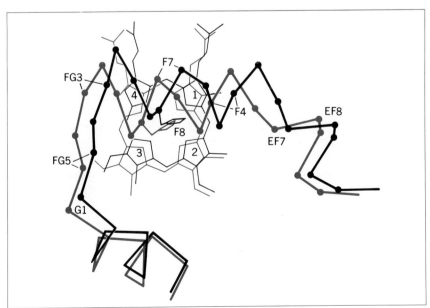

Figure 2.27 Helix and heme motion in the α subunit during the transition between deoxyhemoglobin (black) and carbonmonoxyhemoglobin (color), which is similar to deoxyhemoglobin. Motion in the β subunits is similar, except that the heme also tilts about a ring 2–ring 4 axis, with ring 3 rising out of the plane of the page by 1 Å. (From reference A25.)

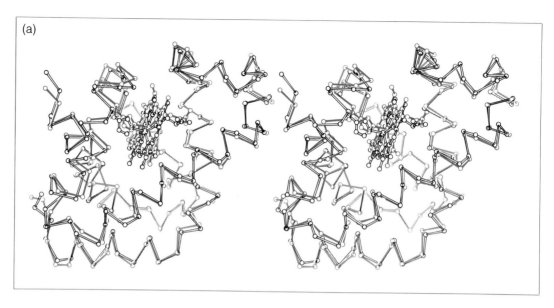

(a)

Figure 2.28 Helix and heme motion in the β subunit. (a) Superposition of heme and main-chain stereos of deoxyhemoglobin (black) and carbonmonoxyhemoglobin (color). Notice the motion of the F helix, the motion and tilt of the heme, and the fadeout of changes halfway along the E and G helices. Note also the shift in the carboxy terminus (upper left) after the freeing of Tyr 145. (Stereo drawing courtesy of T. Takano.)

0.4 Å downward, and sinks 0.6 Å closer to the heme. But in this subunit there is more motion of the heme itself. It shifts 1.0 Å to the left and 1.1 Å deeper into the heme pocket. It also pivots about a diagonal axis through its rings 2 and 4. The vinyl side chain of ring 3 rises 1.0 Å out of the plane of the figure, pushing against Val FG5; ring 1 sinks 0.9 Å into the page toward the E helix. This combination of shifting and twisting moves the ligand binding site away from the side chain of Val E11, which in the β chain blocks access to the heme iron in the deoxy configuration. All of the β-chain motions can be seen in the composite stereo of Figure 2.28a. As with α, most of the heme and F-helix disturbances are dissipated in the E and G helices, leaving the rest of the β subunit little changed.

An important consequence of ligand binding is the beginning of the breakup of the network of hydrogen bonds and salt links at the ends of the molecule. Both the upward shift of the F helix shown in Figure 2.28b, and the contact between heme and the Val FG5 side chain shown in Figure 2.28c, have the effect of weakening and ultimately breaking the hydrogen bond between the Val FG5 carbonyl group and the side chain of Tyr HC2 on the same subunit* (Figure 2.28c). This leads to a loosening of the bonds shown in Figure 2.24 for the subunit that acquires the ligand, making a T-to-R subunit transition easier. Furthermore, the upward shift in the F helix shown in Figure 2.28b cannot take place completely without subunit rearrangement, since in the deoxy or T configuration each FG corner is packed closely against the C helix of an α chain (Figure 2.22). Only after the subunits shift to their oxy or R configuration are the FG corners free to expand in a way that allows total readjustment around the heme, and strainfree binding of the sixth ligand. The movement of the F helix simultaneusly relieves the strain at the heme produced by ligand binding, creates new strain at the FG corner that can only be relieved by a T-to-R subunit shift, and begins the disruption of bonds at the chain termini that makes this shift possible.

---

*For many years it was almost axiomatic in hemoglobin x-ray papers that Tyr HC2 was locked in place by a hydrogen bond to Val FG5 in deoxyhemoglobin but swung free in solution in methemoglobin. This was because the image of the tyrosine and the final residue that followed it was poorly defined in the electron density maps of methemoglobin. In the recent Hemoglobin Atlas, however, the authors have backed away from this all-or-nothing model (7). They now state more cautiously that Tyr HC2 is bound in place in deoxyhemoglobin and is partially delocalized in oxyhemoglobin, spending part of its time free in solution. The red/green stereo drawings, however, show it in its hydrogen-bonded location.

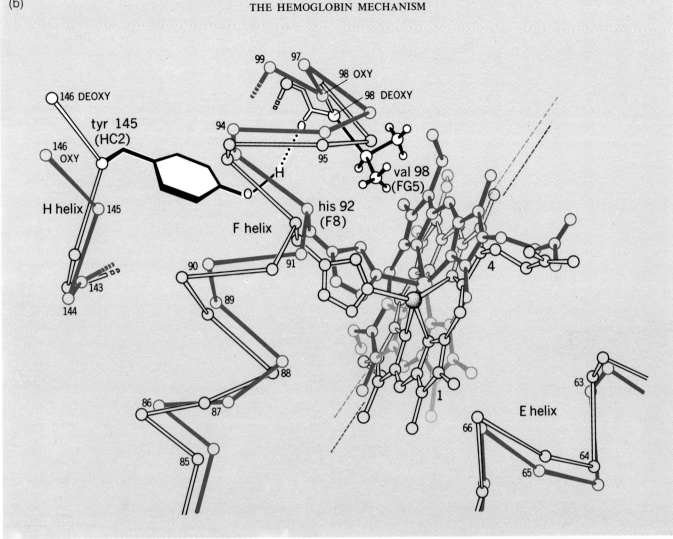

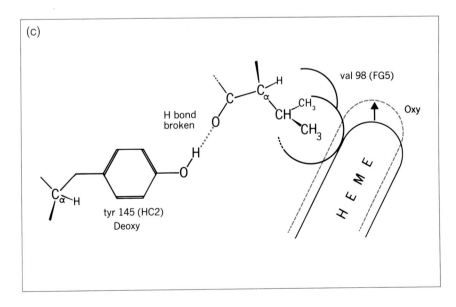

(b) Close-up of the β heme region, with addition of side chains of Val 98(FG5) and Tyr 145(HC2). When the heme tilts in the R conformation (color), the vinyl group of ring 3 pushes against Val 98. The shift from deoxy to carbonmonoxy (or oxy) stretches and weakens the tyrosine hydrogen bond. The propionic acid on ring 1 has been omitted for clarity.

(c) Schematic illustrating the connection between heme motion and tyrosine hydrogen breakage.

There is no reason to regard an unliganded hemoglobin subunit in its deoxy configuration as being strained (27, 28). In fact, resonance Raman spectroscopic measurements of iron–nitrogen stretching frequencies show no indication of strain (29). In this respect the designation T for "tense" is a misnomer. Strain is introduced only when a ligand attempts to bind to a heme that is held in a domed configuration with an out-of-plane iron atom (Figure 2.29a and b). If the FG corners are restricted by contacts with neighboring C helices, then strain must follow either between the heme and the ligand or between the heme and the protein groups on its other side, with the heme adopting an intermediate shape and position that minimizes overall energy. After T-to-R subunit motion, the FG corners can expand freely, the F helix and side chains about the heme can adjust, His F8 can move until it brings the iron atom into the heme plane, and the strain produced by ligand binding once again is relieved (Figure 2.29c). Once the T-to-R transition has been triggered by pressure from the FG corner and weakening of the hydrogen bonds around Tyr HC2, it continues until the side chain of His β97(FG4) is carried to the other side of Thr α41(C6), as shown in Figures 2.20 and 2.21. This ratchet movement of His and Thr past one another probably is of value because it tends to make the subunit transition a two-state, either–or affair, and minimizes the contribution of intermediate states.

Association constants of all the hemes in the T state, A_T, are small because each new ligand bound introduces more strain. The T-to-R transition involves a trade-off of this accumulated strain energy against the energy required to break up the networks of hydrogen bonds and salt links at the top and the bottom of the molecule. If these bonds were not present, then the transition presumably would occur as soon as the first ligand molecule bound. Conversely, without these salt links and hydrogen bonds there would be no reason for an oxyhemoglobin molecule to return to the T configuration at all, even after all four O_2 were gone. The bonds depicted in Figure 2.24 are more than just a source of Bohr protons. They are the springs that bring the partially deoxygenated molecule back into the T conformation and help push away the final O_2 molecules.

2.7 EXPERIMENTAL TESTS

This hemoglobin mechanism not only agrees with theoretical energy calculations but was suggested by them before all the high-resolution x-ray structure refinements had been completed (27, 28). The mechanism also has been tested in ingenious ways using chemically modified or mutant hemoglobins:

1. If a strong ligand such as NO is bound to the heme groups, and the subunits then are driven from the R to the T configuration with IHP, the bonds between iron and the ε nitrogen of His F8 are severely strained by the forcing of liganded hemes into the deoxy geometry. Those in the β subunits are stretched and those in the α subunits are actually broken (30, 31).

2. If cyanide is bound irreversibly to either α or β subunits in the met or ferriheme state, and hybrids of the type $\alpha_2^{CN}\beta_2$ and $\alpha_2\beta_2^{CN}$ are prepared with normal ferroheme or deoxy subunits, then the tetramers spontaneously adopt the R configuration unless forced into the T state by binding of IHP or of inorganic phosphate (32). In the absence of these phosphates, the binding of O_2 to the two deoxy subunits has no effect on the NMR spectrum of the cyanomet hemes. If the subunits are driven to the T state by phosphates before O_2 is added, an effect is observed. This suggests that one type of subunit "sees" what has happened to

(a)

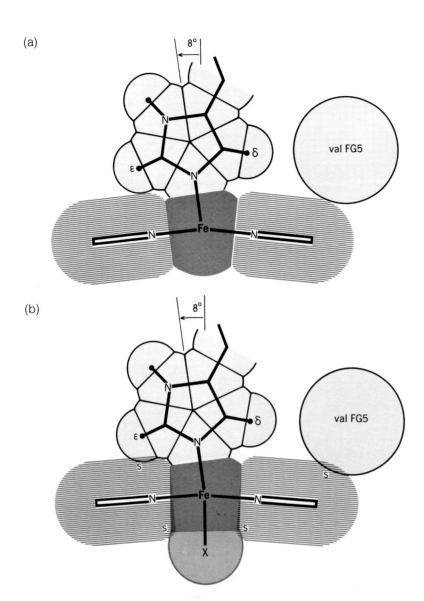

(b)

(c)

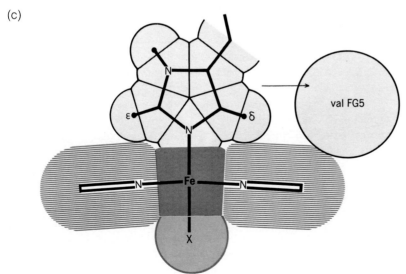

Figure 2.29 Ligation and strain in the heme environment. (a) Unliganded heme in deoxyhemoglobin, with the histidine tilted, the iron out of plane, and the heme in contact with the Val FG5 side chain. (b) Liganded heme held in its deoxy configuration before the T-to-R subunit transition. Steric strain between heme, histidine, ligand, and valine (marked by *s*) can only be relieved after this transition. (c) Relaxed, unstrained liganded heme after the T-to-R shift. Both His F8 and Val FG5 have shifted to the right, and the histidine now is perpendicular to the heme plane. The heme is largely undomed.

the other only via the T-to-R transition, and that subunit reorientation is an essential part of heme–heme cooperativity. In these same cyanomet hybrids, the rate constant for binding CO to hemes increases just when NMR evidence indicates a change from the T to the R state (33), demonstrating that it is the T or R state of the tetramer that determines ligand affinity, not merely the number of ligands already bound.

3. Complementary results are obtained with hemoglobin M Milwaukee,* a mutant in which Val E11 on each β chain is replaced by glutamic acid, with its negative charge stabilizing the met or ferriheme state. This mutant changes from the T to the R subunit arrangement when CO molecules are bound to its two normal α subunits, but the transition can be suppressed by IHP. In the absence of IHP, carbon monoxide binding is cooperative (34) and the binding of CO to the ferrous α hemes produces changes in the near-infrared and magnetic resonance spectra of the ferric β hemes (35, 36). If IHP is present to prevent the T-to-R transition, then no effects are observed.

4. If the carboxy-terminal residues of the α or β chains are removed, then hemoglobin remains in the oxy or R configuration even in the absence of ligands (14), emphasizing the importance of the "springs" at the top and the bottom of the molecule in bringing the tetramer back into the T state. This chain-truncated molecule shows no heme–heme cooperativity and has a hyperbolic oxygen-binding curve like that of myoglobin. It also has a high oxygen affinity, which is comparable to that of myoglobin, isolated hemoglobin subunits, and the last O_2 to bind to normal hemoglobin.

5. A mutant hemoglobin Philly, which has Phe for Tyr at position 35(C1) on each β chain, has been shown by proton NMR to remain in the R state even after losing its oxygens, unless it is pushed into the T state by the binding of IHP (37). Without IHP, hemoglobin Philly binds oxygen noncooperatively and with high affinity. The binding of IHP shifts the molecule to the T state, lowers its oxygen affinity, and induces heme–heme cooperativity.

6. Conversely, mutant hemoglobins that can be induced to retain their T conformation even with four liganding oxygen molecules show no heme–heme cooperativity. They also show an oxygen-binding curve that is hyperbolic like that of myoglobin but shifted to lower O_2 affinity, like that of the first oxygen binding to the T configuration of normal hemoglobin (A14).

All of these studies support the idea that the reduced oxygen affinity of deoxyhemoglobin arises from the T conformation with its cramped FG corners and out-of-plane iron atoms, and that heme–heme cooperativity in ligand binding is associated with the transition between T and R subunit arrangements. Which comes first—the breaking of hydrogen bonds and salt bridges at the top and the bottom of the molecule, or the T-to-R subunit transition? Are the bonds ruptured by the motion of subunits, or is this motion only possible because the bonds stabilizing the T state have been broken first?

The balance of evidence favors the idea that the bonds (shown in Figure 2.24) begin to weaken and rupture as soon as the first O_2 binds to the subunits. It has long been known that the initial release of Bohr protons takes place simultaneously with binding of CO to hemoglobin, even before the T-to-R

---

*Abnormal human hemoglobins that are discovered by routine blood sampling are customarily named after the place in which they are first encountered. These mutant hemoglobins are considered in more detail in Chapter 4.

subunit transition (38, 39). Moreover, breaking the Bohr group salt bridges by pH change or chemical modification alters A_T, the affinity constant of heme for O_2 in the T state (40). By the principle of microreversibility, the binding of ligand to heme should weaken these same salt bridges. Proton NMR studies also indicate that, as hemoglobin picks up oxygen, the hydrogen bond between the penultimate Tyr β145(HC2) and the carbonyl group of Val β97(FG5) breaks before the hydrogen bond between Tyr α42(C7) and Asp β99(G1) does, or that some bonds within a subunit are broken prior to bonds between subunits (41). Hence, in the allosteric equilibrium equation of page 48, states T_1 and T_2 are more than simply the T_0 state with one and two bound oxygens; they represent actual structural intermediates, with certain of the original T_0 bonds strained or broken. Real-time experimental methods such as NMR can detect such states, whereas x-ray analyses of the limiting structures cannot.

In some unusual circumstances, the T state can be locked down so tightly that ligation of the hemes produces neither a T-to-R transition nor a disruption of the bonds at the ends of the chains. The mutant known as hemoglobin Kansas lacks one of the hydrogen bonds stabilizing the R state because Asn β102(G4) is replaced by Thr. Inositol hexaphosphate in solution, and the forces between packed molecules in crystals of the protein, are each enough to freeze hemoglobin Kansas in the T state even after ligands bind to the heme. In both cases the bonds involved in the Bohr effect are found to remain unbroken (42, 43). It was thought at first that this indicated that these bonds were only broken after the T-to-R subunit motion. Actually, it only demonstrates that, with the proper constraints, low-affinity ligand binding can occur in this abnormal hemoglobin molecule without inevitably touching off either bond rupture at the ends or subunit motion. Normal hemoglobin behaves differently.

Which subunits bind oxygen first in normal hemoglobin, α or β? This has not yet been answered satisfactorily. It has been assumed for a long time that the α chains probably bind O_2 more easily, because the binding pocket in β is blocked by the side chain of Val β67(E11). The side chain swings out of the way in oxyhemoglobin, and the tilting of the heme during the T-to-R transition that is characteristic of the β chain but not of the α chain (see Figure 2.28) moves the ligand-binding site on the iron atom away from the E11 side chain. It seemed more reasonable to assume that O_2 bound first to the unobstructed α hemes, and that the β sites were opened up by the T-to-R subunit transition (44). Laser photolysis spectroscopy and other kinetic experiments have shown that one type of heme has three to four times the oxygen affinity of the other in normal deoxyhemoglobin, unfortunately without revealing which is which (45).

2.8   THE HEMOGLOBIN MECHANISM

All of the x-ray, NMR, spectroscopic, chemical, and theoretical evidence just described has led to a reasonably straightforward picture of the hemoglobin mechanism. This mechanism is likely to be correct in principle, even if specific details have to be modified later. Deoxyhemoglobin is held in its T subunit configuration mainly by a network of hydrogen bonds and salt bridges that connect the amino- and carboxy-terminal regions of both chains. In the absence of ligands, the four hemes are in a relaxed, essentially strain-free environment with His F8 tilted off-axis, the heme plane domed toward the His, and an out-of-plane iron atom (Figure 2.29). Strain is produced when a ligand binds on the other side of the heme, and this strain is transmitted through side chains and the F helix to the FG corners and to the terminal salt and hydrogen bonds. Some of these bonds are ruptured, and others are strained. When the strain of ligand binding in the T state becomes great enough (after the second or third ligand is bound), the molecule shifts from the T to the R subunit conformation. This relieves the strain on the already liganded hemes. It also allows the unliganded hemes a potential freedom of motion that enhances their affinity for oxygen, facilitating the total oxygenation of the hemoglobin molecule. In the reverse cycle, removing one or more O_2 from the molecule in the R configuration does not necessarily introduce any new strain, but it lowers the energy barrier against a shift to the T state and a re-formation of the terminal salt and hydrogen bonds. When the stability that this bond re-formation would produce becomes greater than the energy required to force the remaining liganded hemes into the tilted histidine, T-like conformation, the switch from R to T occurs. The strain introduced by the subunit transition can be relieved by ejecting the remaining O_2 molecules, so their release is accomplished more easily. Although the T-to-R transition is not a rigid, all-or-nothing event (no macromolecular processes are), it can be treated conveniently in the framework of the allosteric theory. DPG, protons, chloride ions, and carbon dioxide all act as allosteric effectors, favoring the deoxy or T state.

Figure 2.30 The switch region of the $\alpha_1\beta_2$ interface and its symmetrical twin, $\alpha_2\beta_1$, are highlighted in a top view of oxyhemoglobin. Evolutionarily invariant residues that are visible in this top view are shown by color dots. See Figures 2.20 and 3.2 for more details.

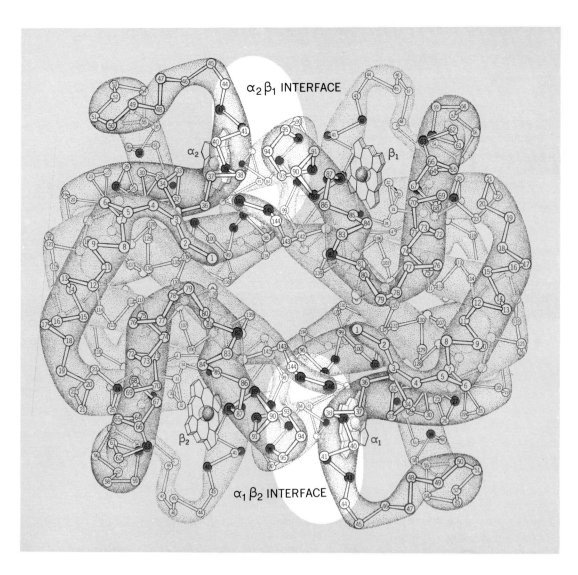

If hemoglobin is regarded as a molecular machine, the engine room in retrospect seems to be the $\alpha_1\beta_2$ interface. This region, seen in Figure 2.22, contains both the flexible joint and the switch. It also contains the penultimate tyrosine whose loosening is an early step in the T to R transition, and most of the groups implicated in the Bohr effect. Figure 2.30 shows the switch region of $\alpha_1\beta_2$ as well as the $\alpha_2\beta_1$ interface, along with the concentration of evolutionarily invariant positions among all known vertebrates. Akers and coworkers have found that most of the free energy difference between T and R states is localized in the $\alpha_1\beta_2$ interface (47); in some cases, alteration of only a single amino acid can destroy this free energy difference. It will come as no surprise, therefore, to find in the next chapter that the $\alpha_1\beta_2$ interface is one of the most strongly conserved regions of the molecule throughout evolutionary history. And finally, the mutant studies considered in Chapter 4 show that amino acid substitutions in this critical interface invariably lead to abnormal behavior and often to serious pathologies.

How did such a complex and beautifully constructed molecular machine develop? This is the subject of the next chapter, on molecular evolution.

GENERAL REFERENCES

1. Lehninger, A. L., 1975. *Biochemistry* (2nd ed.), Worth, New York.
2. White, A., Handler, P., Smith, E. L., Hill, R. L., and Lehman, I. R., 1978. *Principles of Biochemistry* (6th ed.), McGraw-Hill, New York.
3. Stryer, L., 1981. *Biochemistry* (2nd Ed.), Freeman, San Francisco.
4. Lehmann, H., and Huntsman, R. G., 1974. *Man's Haemoglobins* (2nd ed.), North-Holland Publishing Company, Amsterdam.
5. Antonini, E., and Brunori, M., 1971. *Hemoglobin and Myoglobin in Their Reactions with Ligands,* North-Holland Publishing Company, Amsterdam.
6. Wood, W. G., Old, J. M., Roberts, A. V. S., Clegg, J. B., Weatherall, D. J., and Quattrin, N., 1978. *Cell* 15:437–446.
7. Perutz, M. F., and Fermi, G., 1981. *Haemoglobin and Myoglobin,* Atlas of Molecular Structures in Biology, Vol. 2, Oxford University Press, New York.
8. Bernal, J. D., Fankuchen, I., and Perutz, M. F., 1938. *Nature* 141:523–524.
9. Perutz, M. F., Rossmann, M. G., Cullis, A. F., Muirhead, H., Will, G., and North, A. C. T., 1960. *Nature* 185:416–422.
10. Dayhoff, M. O. *Atlas of Protein Sequence and Structure:* Vol. 5 (1972); Supplement 1 (1973); Supplement 2 (1976); Supplement 3 (1978). Georgetown University, Washington, D.C. (All earlier volumes are superseded by Vol. 5 and its supplements.)
11. Croft, L. R., 1973. *Handbook of Protein Sequences,* Joynson-Bruvvers, Oxford.
12. Fasman, G. D., 1976. *Handbook of Biochemistry and Molecular Biology: Proteins Series,* Vol. 3, CRC Press, Cleveland.
13. Chothia, C., Janin, J., and Wodak, S., 1976. *Proc. Natl. Acad. Sci. USA* 73:3793–3797.
14. Kilmartin, J. V., and Rossi-Bernardi, L., 1973. *Physiol. Rev.* 53:836–890.
15. Kilmartin, J. V., 1976. *Brit. Med. Bull.* 32:209–212.
16. Nishikura, K., 1978. *Biochem. J.* 173:671–675.
17. Perutz, M. F., Kilmartin, J. V., Nishikura, K., Fogg, J. R., Butler, P. J. G., and Rollema, H. S., 1980. *J. Mol. Biol.* 138:649–670.

18. Russu, I. M., Ho, N. T., and Ho, C. 1980. *Biochemistry* 19:1043–1052.
19. Matthew, J. B., Hanania, G. I. H., and Gurd, F. R. N., 1979. *Biochemistry* 18:1928–1936; Matthew, J. B., Friend, S. H. and Gurd, F. R. N., 1981. *Biochemistry* 20:571–580.
20. Perutz, M. F., and Imai, K., 1980. *J. Mol. Biol.* 136:183–191.
21. Bonaventura, J., Bonaventura, C., Amiconi, G., Tentori, L., Brunori, M., and Antonini, E., 1975. *J. Biol. Chem.* 250:6278–6281.
22. Monod, J., Wyman, J., and Changeux, J. P., 1965. *J. Mol. Biol.* 12:88–118.
23. Shulman, R. G., Hopfield, J. J., and Ogawa, S., 1975. *Quart. Rev. Biophys.* 8:325–420.
24. Baldwin, J. M., 1976. *Brit. Med. Bull.* 32:213–218.
25. MacQuarrie, R., and Gibson, Q. H., 1972. *J. Biol. Chem.* 247:5686–5694.
26. Eisenberger, P., Shulman, R. G., Kincaid, B. M., Brown, G. S., and Ogawa, S., 1978. *Nature* 274:30–34.
27. Gelin, B. R., and Karplus, M., 1977. *Proc. Natl. Acad. Sci. USA* 74:801–805.
28. Warshel, A., 1977. *Proc. Natl. Acad. Sci. USA* 74:1789–1793.
29. Kincaid, J., Stein, P., and Spiro, T. G., 1979. *Proc. Natl. Acad. Sci. USA* 76:549–552.
30. Perutz, M. F., Kilmartin, J. V., Nagai, K., Szabo, A., and Simon, S. R., 1976. *Biochemistry* 15:378–387.
31. Maxwell, J. C., and Caughey, W. S., 1976. *Biochemistry* 15:388–396.
32. Ogawa, S., and Shulman, R. G., 1972. *J. Mol. Biol.* 70:315–336.
33. Cassoly, R., Gibson, Q. H., Ogawa, S., and Shulman, R. G., 1971. *Biochem. Biophys. Res. Commun.* 44:1015–1021.
34. Udem, L., Ranney, H. M., Bunn, H. F., and Pisciotta, A., 1970. *J. Mol. Biol.* 48:489–498.
35. Lindstrom, T. R., Ho, C., and Pisciotta, A. V., 1972. *Nature New Biol.* 237:263–264.
36. Perutz, M. F., Pulsinelli, P. S., and Ranney, H. M., 1972. *Nature New Biol.* 237:259–263.
37. Asakura, T., Adachi, K., Wiley, J. S., Fung, L. W.-M., Ho, C., Kilmartin, J. V., and Perutz, M. F., 1976. *J. Mol. Biol.* 104:185–195.
38. Antonini, E., Schuster, T. M., Brunori, M., and Wyman, J., 1965. *J. Biol. Chem.* 240:PC2262–PC2264.
39. Gray, R. D., 1970. *J. Biol. Chem.* 245:2914–2921.
40. Kilmartin, J. V., Imai, K., Jones, R. T., Faruqui, A. R., Fogg, J., and Baldwin, J. M., 1978. *Biochim. Biophys. Acta* 534:15–25.
41. Viggiano, G., and Ho, C., 1979. *Proc. Natl. Acad. Sci. USA* 76:3673–3677.
42. Anderson, L., 1975. *J. Mol. Biol.* 94:33–49.
43. Kilmartin, J. V., Anderson, N. L., and Ogawa, S., 1978. *J. Mol. Biol.* 123:71–87.
44. Perutz, M. F., 1970. *Nature* 228:726–739.
45. Sawicki, C. A., and Gibson, Q. H., 1977. *J. Biol. Chem.* 252:7538–7547.
46. Perutz, M. F., Hasnain, S. S., Duke, P. J., Sessler, J. L., and Hahn, J. E., 1982. *Nature* 295:535–538.
47. Pettigrew, D. W., Romeo, P. H., Tsapis, A., Thillet, J., Smith, M. L., Turner, B. W., and Ackers, G. K., 1982. *Proc. Natl. Acad. Sci.* 79:1849–1853.
48. Ladner, R. C., Air, G. M., and Fogg, J. H., 1976. *J. Mol. Biol.* 103:675–677.

APPENDIX

APPENDIX 2.1   VERTEBRATE GLOBIN STRUCTURE ANALYSES

This appendix lists all the structure analyses of normal vertebrate myoglobins and tetrameric hemoglobins that, at the time of writing, had been carried to the point where a complete polypeptide chain path could be traced unambiguously. Structure analyses of monomeric globins are listed after Chapter 3, and abnormal hemoglobins after Chapter 4. The date in the first column is not the year in which research was begun, or a high-resolution map was first calculated. Rather, it is the year in which the first refereed journal publication appeared containing complete information about the protein chain tracing at high resolution. Molecular weights of individual subunits are given, including heme groups. Numbers of subunits are indicated outside the parentheses. Molecular weights based on amino acid sequences are given with full significant figures, but approximate molecular weights from physical measurements are given in thousands: "13K" means roughly 13,000. Amino acids are listed on a per-subunit basis, and the number of each type of subunit is not indicated. The column marked "Analysis" gives the state of the crystal-structure analysis at time of writing: first the resolution in angstroms, and then a brief description of the method. For this, MIR = multiple isomorphous replacement; SIR = single isomorphous replacement; Ano = anomalous scattering data; Mol. = molecular-replacement methods using coordinates taken from some related structure; $\Delta F \ \phi_{xx}$ = difference-map analysis using phases from structure analysis xx; Ref. = true crystallographic refinement by real-space, difference-map, or least-squares methods, followed by the percent residual error or R factor. Only a small number of key references have been included, usually the first paper to establish the polypeptide chain path and the most recent papers that provide entries into the earlier literature.

Date	Protein	Source	Mol. Wt.	Amino Acids	Analysis	Refs.
1960	Myoglobin, met	Sperm whale	17,815	153	2.0 Ref. 23.5%	A1–4
1966	Myoglobin, deoxy	Sperm whale	17,815	153	2.0 Ref. 23.5%	A5,6
1978	Myoglobin, oxy	Sperm whale	17,815	153	2.0 Ref. 20%	A7
1975	Myoglobin, CO	Sperm whale	17,815	153	1.8 ΔF, ϕ_{met}	A8
1964	Myoglobin, azo	Sperm whale	17,815	153	2.0 ΔF, ϕ_{met}	A9
1978	Myoglobin, met	Seal	17,913	153	2.5 MIR	A10
1968	Hemoglobin, met	Horse	2(15,730) + 2(16,595)	141/146	2.0 Ref 23.1%	A11–15
1970	Hemoglobin, deoxy	Horse	2(15,730) + 2(15,595)	141/146	2.8 MIR	A15,16
1970	Hemoglobin, deoxy	Man	2(15,742) + 2(16,483)	141/146	2.5 Ref. 28.8%	A17–19
1975	Hemoglobin, deoxy (from PEG)	Man	2(15,742) + 2(16,483)	141/146	3.5 Mol.	A20
1972	Hemoglobin, deoxy/DPG or IHP	Man	2(15,742) + 2(16,483)	141/146	3.5 ΔF, ϕ_{deoxy}	A21,22
1977	Hemoglobin, fetal deoxy	Man	2(15,742) + 2(15,593)	141/146	2.5 SIR + Mol	A23
1976	Hemoglobin, CO	Horse	2(15,730) + 2(16,595)	141/146	2.8 ΔF, ϕ_{met}	A24
1979	Hemoglobin, CO	Man	2(15,742) + 2(15,593)	141/146	2.8	A25
1976	Hemoglobin, CN⁻ met	Horse	2(15,730) + 2(16,595)	141/146	2.8 ΔF, ϕ_{met}	A26
1976	Hemoglobin, F⁻ met	Horse	2(15,730) + 2(16,595)	141/146	2.8 ΔF, ϕ_{met}	A27
1976	Hemoglobin, F⁻ met + IHP	Man	2(15,742) + 2(16,483)	141/146	3.5 ΔF, ϕ_{deoxy}	A28
1976	Hemoglobin, met mangano	Horse	2(15,730) + 2(16,595)	141/146	2.8 ΔF, ϕ_{met}	A29
1976	Hemoglobin, deuteroheme	Horse	2(15,730) + 2(16,595)	141/146	2.8 ΔF, ϕ_{met}	A30
1977	Hemoglobin, mesoheme	Horse	2(15,730) + 2(16,595)	141/146	2.8 ΔF, ϕ_{met}	A31
1979	Hemoglobin, NO	Horse	2(15,730) + 2(16,595)	141/146	2.8 ΔF, ϕ_{met}	A32
1979	Hemoglobin, azo	Horse	2(15,730) + 2(16,595)	141/146	2.8 ΔF, ϕ_{met}	A33
1981	Hemoglobin H (β_4)	Man	4(16,483)	146	2.5 Ref. 20%	A34

For other abnormal human hemoglobins, see Chapter 4.

GLASSES FOR VIEWING STEREO DRAWINGS

Simple, inexpensive cardboard viewers with magnifying lenses for viewing stereo pair drawings are available from Taylor Merchant Corporation, 212 West 35th Street, New York, New York 10001. Materials are also available for viewing and projecting stereo slides.

A more durable plastic viewer with cast-plastic lenses and a wire stand (model number 575) may be purchased from Hubbard Scientific Company, Box 105, Northbrook, Illinois 60062.

Professional metal viewers with accurately ground lenses may be obtained from Abrams Instrument Corporation, 606 East Shiawassee Street, Lansing, Michigan 48912.

HEMOGLOBIN MODEL SYSTEMS

An inexpensive preassembled hemoglobin model with separate color-coded side chains is available from Vis-Aid Devices, 857 Mulvey Avenue, Winnipeg, Manitoba R3M 1G6, Canada.

Professional hemoglobin models are built to order from functionally color-coded polyethylene units at a scale of 1 cm per Angstrom by John Mack, Apt. 8B, 66 Overlook Terrace, New York, New York 10040.

A complete hemoglobin molecule is available as a model kit or preassembled structure using a system of precisely set torsion angles. This framework model (convertible to space-filling) is available from Academic Press, 111 Fifth Avenue, New York, New York 10003.

APPENDIX 2.1 REFERENCES

A1. Kendrew, J. C., Dickerson, R. E., Strandberg, B. E., Hart, R. G., Davies, D. R., Phillips, D. C., and Shore, V. C., 1960. *Nature* 185:422–427.

A2. Kendrew, J. C., 1961. *Scientific American* (December):96–110.

A3. Watson, H. C., 1969. *Prog. Stereochem.* 4:299–333.

A4. Takano, T., 1977. *J. Mol. Biol.* 110:537–568.

A5. Nobbs, C. L., Watson, H. C., and Kendrew, J. C., 1966. *Nature* 209:339–341.

A6. Takano, T., 1977. *J. Mol. Biol.* 110:569–584.

A7. Phillips, S. E. V., 1978. *Nature* 273:247–248.

A8. Norvell, J. C., Nunes, A. C., and Schoenborn, B. P., 1975. *Science* 190:568–569.

A9. Stryer, L., Kendrew, J. C., and Watson, H. C., 1964. *J. Mol. Biol.* 8:96–104.

A10. Scouloudi, H., and Baker, E. N., 1978. *J. Mol. Biol.* 126:637–660.

A11. Perutz, M. F., 1964. *Scientific American* (November):64–76.

A12. Perutz, M. F., Muirhead, H., Cox, J. M., and Goaman, L. C. G., 1968. *Nature* 219:131–139.

A13. Ladner, R. C., Heidner, E. J., and Perutz, M. F., 1977. *J. Mol. Biol.* 114:385–414.

A14. Perutz, M. F., 1978. *Scientific American* (December):92–125.

A15. Perutz, M. F., 1979. *Ann. Rev. Bioch.* 48:327–386.

A16. Bolton, W., and Perutz, M. F., 1970. *Nature* 228:551–552.

A17. Muirhead, H., and Greer, J., 1970. *Nature* 228:516–519.

A18. Fermi, G., 1975. *J. Mol. Biol.* 97:237–256.

A19. Ten Eyck, L. F., and Arnone, A., 1976. *J. Mol. Biol.* 100:3–11.

A20. Ward, K. B., Wishner, B. C., Lattman, E. E., and Love, W. E., 1975. *J. Mol. Biol.* 90:161–177.

A21. Arnone, A., 1972. *Nature* 237:146–149.

A22. Arnone, A., and Perutz, M. F., 1974. *Nature* 249:34–36.

A23. Frier, J. A., and Perutz, M. F., 1977. *J. Mol. Biol.* 112:97–112.

A24. Heidner, E. J., Ladner, R. C., and Perutz, M. F., 1976. *J. Mol. Biol.* 104:707–722.

A25. Baldwin, J., and Chothia, C., 1979. *J. Mol. Biol.* 129:175–220.

A26. Deatherage, J. F., Loe, R. S., Anderson, C. M., and Moffat, K., 1976. *J. Mol. Biol.* 104:687–706.

A27. Deatherage, J. F., Loe, R. S., and Moffat, K., 1976. *J. Mol. Biol.* 104:723–728.

A28. Fermi, G., and Perutz, M. F., 1977. *J. Mol. Biol.* 114:421–431.

A29. Moffat, K., Loe, R. S., and Hoffman, B. M., 1976. *J. Mol. Biol.* 104:669–685.

A30. Seybert, D. W., and Moffat, K., 1976. *J. Mol. Biol.* 106:895–903.

A31. Seybert, D. W., and Moffat, K., 1977. *J. Mol. Biol.* 113:419–430.

A32. Deatherage, J. F., and Moffat, K., 1979. *J. Mol. Biol.* 134:401–417.

A33. Deatherage, J. F, Obendorf, S. K., and Moffat, K., 1979. *J. Mol. Biol.* 134:419–429.

A34. Arnone, A., Briley, P. D., and Rogers, P. H., in press. In C. Ho (Ed.), *Interactions between Iron and Proteins in Oxygen and Electron Transport,* Elsevier North Holland, New York.

EXON-CODED DOMAINS IN HEMOGLOBIN

Each hemoglobin gene, no matter what type, contains three exons, or regions of DNA that ultimately will be translated into amino acid sequences, separated by two introns, or nontranslated DNA regions. Introns are transcribed into messenger RNA, and then edited out of the message before it is used at the ribosomes. The breaks separating exon-coded domains occur at precisely the same places in all hemoglobin chains: between residues B12 and B13, and between G6 and G7, arguing for a great antiquity and a common evolutionary origin for the exon–intron gene organization. Each exon-coded domain has its own structural role in the folded protein. Exon 1 builds the A and B helices (upper left), which form a scaffolding for the heme pockets and the sliding contacts in the complete tetramer. The long exon 2 domain (lower left) provides the heme pocket (E and F helices) and the $\alpha_1\beta_2$ sliding contacts (C helix and FG corner). Exon 3 contributes the G and H helices, including most of the $\alpha_1\beta_1$ packing contacts. Two side views of the hemoglobin tetramer at upper and lower right show this third exon product during the oxy–deoxy subunit transition. In primitive monomeric leghemoglobin, exon 2 is interrupted between codons for residues E14 and E15 (dashed line) by yet another intron, which may have been lost by the higher hemoglobin genes.

3 EVOLUTION OF THE OXYGEN CARRIERS

CHAPTER 3

EVOLUTION OF
THE OXYGEN CARRIERS

The idea that macromolecules have an evolutionary history fully as traceable as that of bone structure or any other large-scale feature developed on the heels of the first determinations of amino acid sequences of proteins: bovine insulin in 1951 (1, 2); other small peptide hormones in subsequent years; horse cytochrome c (3) and the α and β chains of horse hemoglobin (4) in 1961; and bovine ribonuclease (5), hen egg white lysozyme (6), and bovine chymotrypsinogen (7) in 1963. Anfinsen's monograph, *The Molecular Basis of Evolution* (8), is a classic that can be read with profit even though it first appeared in 1959.

The structural side of the study of macromolecular evolution began in the fall of 1959, when Perutz and his team of protein crystallographers in Cambridge examined the low-resolution model of horse methemoglobin (9). They realized that each of its four chains was folded exactly like the chain seen in the parallel high-resolution structure analysis of sperm whale myoglobin that had just been completed by Kendrew and co-workers in the same laboratory (10). The amino acid sequences were still unknown, and raw amino acid composition comparisons did not suggest a great similarity of structure. If any casual laboratory conversations were held prior to these x-ray results, suggesting that the myoglobin and hemoglobin chains might be folded identically, these have vanished from memory. It therefore was a genuine surprise, and a trigger for evolutionary thinking, to see in late 1959 that hemoglobin was "just four myoglobin molecules put together." As Perutz expressed it in the first low-resolution hemoglobin paper (9),

> How does this arise? It is scarcely conceivable that a three-dimensional template forces the chain to take up this fold. More probably the chain, once it is synthesized and provided with a haem group around which it can coil, takes up this configuration spontaneously, as the only one which satisfies the stereochemical requirements of its amino acid sequence. This suggests the occurrence of similar sequences throughout this group of proteins, despite their marked differences in amino acid content. This seems all the more likely, since their structural similarity suggests that they have developed from a common genetic precursor.

Once the amino acid sequences of hemoglobin and myoglobin were available, they confirmed Perutz' intuition—the chains are so similar that they must have shared a common ancestral gene (4, 11). The history of the globin family evidently was one of duplication of an original gene coding for an oxygen-binding globin molecule, followed by the independent accumulation of mutations leading to present-day sequence differences in myoglobin and hemoglobin chains, as diagrammed in Figure 3.1.

3.1 GLOBIN SEQUENCE COMPARISONS

The two decades following the initial globin sequence analyses saw the determination of at least 60 different α family (α, ζ) sequences from vertebrates ranging from shark and carp to viper and man, 66 sequences of the β family (β, γ, δ, ε), and 60 myoglobins (see Appendix 3.2). In addition, 11 single-chain globin sequences have been obtained from two kinds of lamprey, from invertebrates such as shellfish, marine worms, and insect larva, and from the root nodules of legumes such as soybean, kidney bean, and yellow lupine. These sequences make up the largest body of information on comparative molecular evolution available for any one family of proteins, with only the c-type cytochromes as competition.

A representative selection of globin sequences is given in Table 3.1. These sequences have been chosen to illustrate the main points that can be learned from the full set of data. Other sequences can be found in the Dayhoff *Atlas* and its supplements (12), and in an excellent review by Thompson (13). The sequences chosen for Table 3.1 include those for a few placental mammals, one monotreme (platypus), one bird (chicken), and where known, one bony fish (carp) and one cartilaginous fish (Port Jackson shark). The monomeric globins selected include those of lamprey, one shellfish (the mollusc *Aplysia*), the marine bloodworm *Glycera dibranchiata,* the larva of the midge *Chironomus thummii,* and two leghemoglobins from the root nodules of legumes.

Each of the three main families of globin chains—α, β, and myoglobin—has its own particular pattern of similarities. The light color bars in Table 3.1 denote amino acid residues that are identical in *all* known sequences of a given family, not just those shown in the table. All 60 known α hemoglobin chains have identical amino acids at 23 of their 141 positions. All 66 known β-family chains have identical residues at 20 of their 146 positions, and the 60 known myoglobin sequences are identical at 27 of their 153 positions. If only mammals are compared, of course, then there are more identical positions (short bars in Table 3.1): 50 for the α family, 51 for the β family, and 71—nearly half—for myoglobins. Hemoglobin invariants for α and β chains are mapped on pages 70 and 71, and myoglobin invariants on page 72.

Looking only at amino acid identities is too restrictive from a functional standpoint. Many positions in Table 3.1 are uncolored only because an arginine has been substituted for a lysine in one or two species, or a leucine for isoleucine. Similar residues often can do the same job, and if we were to include positions where one residue has been replaced by a functionally equivalent one, then many more positions would be colored. This can be appreciated by turning back to Table 2.3, which gives the identities in whale myoglobin and horse and human hemoglobins, and seeing what other residues now are encountered at these positions if one examines all 186 of the vertebrate globin chains, as can be seen in Table 3.2 at the top of page 73. Five positions remain totally invariant, and the ones that change generally do so to another side chain of similar properties. The underlined residue in each case is by far the dominant choice; the alternatives

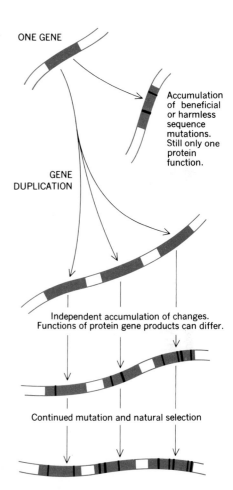

ONE GENE

Accumulation of beneficial or harmless sequence mutations. Still only one protein function.

GENE DUPLICATION

Independent accumulation of changes. Functions of protein gene products can differ.

Continued mutation and natural selection

GENES FOR RELATED BUT DISTINCT PROTEINS

Figure 3.1 Evolution through gene duplication. Diversification of enzymes or other gene products and evolution of new proteins can only occur through multiple gene copies. If at least one of the copies is still making the original protein, then the others can accumulate mutations that lead to new or modified functions. In this way the myoglobin and α, β, γ, δ, ε, and ζ hemoglobin genes evolved from those of a common ancestral globin.

usually are encountered in one, two, or a handful of species. Significant alterations in the nature of a side chain occur at only five positions—A12, A14, A15, E5, and FG2—and for one species each. Even these differences probably imply only local alterations in protein folding. Ser A12 and Asp A15 can sit inside a protein if they are hydrogen bonded to a polar group such as a main-chain C=O or N—H. Leu E5 can be tucked out of the way between the B and E helices, and Ile FG2 sits on the edge of the heme pocket.

TABLE 3.1 SEQUENCE COMPARISONS WITHIN THE GLOBIN FAMILY

HELIX NOTATION	A1	A8	AB1	B4	B12	C1	C4	CD1	D1	E1	E8	E15

ALPHA HEMOGLOBIN CHAIN (60 sequences; 23 invariant residues)

```
                 1 2 3 4 5 6 7 8 9 10 11 12 13 14 15 16 17 18 19 20 21 22 23   24 25 26 27 28 29 30 31 32 33 34 35 36 37 38 39 40 41 42 43 44 45 46   47 48 49 50   51 52 53 54 55 56 57 58 59 60 61 62 63   64 65 66 67
α Man ............ V—L S P A D K T N V K A A W G K V G A H A G E——Y G A E A L E R M F L S F P T T K T Y F P H F—D L S H———————G S A Q V K G H G K K V A—D A L T
α Rhesus monkey .. V—L S P A D K S N V K A A W G K V G G H A G E——Y G A E A L E R M F L S F P T T K T Y F P H F—D L S H———————G S A Q V K G H G K K V A—D A L T
α Cow ............ V—L S A A D K G N V K A A W G K V G G H A A E——Y G A E A L E R M F L S F P T T K T Y F P H F—D L S H———————G S A Q V K G H G A K V A—A A L T
α Platypus ....... M—L T D A E K K E V T A L W G K A A G H G E E——Y G A E A L E R L F Q A F P T T K T Y F S H F—D L S H———————G S A Q I K A H G K K V A—D A L S
α Chicken ........ V—L S N A D K N N V K G I F T K I A G H A E E——Y G A E T L E R M F I G F P T T K T Y F P H F—D L S H———————G S A Q I K G H G K K V A—L A I T
ζ Man ............ S—L T K T Q R T I I V S M W A K I S T Q A D T——I G T E T L E R L F L S H P Q T K T Y F P H F—D L H P———————G S R E L R A H G S K V V—A A V G
α Carp ........... S—L S D K D K A A V K I A W A K I S P K A D D——I G A E A L G R M L T V Y P Q A T K S Y F K H W A D L S P———————G S G P V K—H G K K V I M G A V G
α Shark S T S T S T S D—Y S A A D R A E L A A L S K V L A Q N A E A——F G A E A L A R M F T V Y A A K S Y F K D Y K D F T A———————A A P S I K A H G A K V V—T A L A
                                                            π    π π σ σ  σ σ σ  σ
                                                            T        T    T
```

BETA HEMOGLOBIN CHAIN (66 sequences; 20 invariant residues)

```
                 1 2 3 4 5 6 7 8 9 10 11 12 13 14 15 16 17 18   19 20 21 22   23 24 25 26 27 28 29 30 31 32 33 34 35 36 37   38 39 40 41   42 43 44 45 46 47 48 49 50 51 52 53 54 55 56 57 58 59 60 61 62 63 64 65 66 67 68   69 70 71 72
β Rhesus monkey .. V H L T P E E K N A V T T L W G K V——N V D E——V G G E A L G R L L L V V Y P W T Q R F F E S F G D L S S P D A V M G N P K V K A H G K K V L—G A F S
β Man ............ V H L T P E E K S A V T A L W G K V——N V D E——V G G E A L G R L L V V Y P W T Q R F F E S F G D L S T P D A V M G N P K V K A H G K K V L—G A F S
δ Man ............ V H L T P E E K T A V N A L W G K V——N V D A——V G G E A L G R L L V V Y P W T Q R F F E S F G D L S S P D A V M G N P K V K A H G K K V L—G A F S
β Cow ............ M—L T A E E K A A V T A F W S K V——H V D E——V G G E A L G R L L V V Y P W T Q R F F E S F G D L S T A D A V M D N P K V K A H G K K V L—D S F S
"γ" Cow (Fetal β) M—L S A E E K A A V T S L F A K V——K V D E——V G G E A L G R L L V V Y P W T Q R F F E S F G D L S S A D A I L G N P K V K A H G K K V L—D S F C
γ Man ............ G H F T E E D K A T I T S L W G K V——N V E D——A G G E T L G R L L V V Y P W T Q R F F D S F G N L S S A S A I M G N P K V K A H G K K V L—T S L G
ε Man ............ V H F T A E E K S A V T S L W S K M——N V E E——A G G E A L G R L L V V Y P W T Q R F F D S F G N L S S P S A I L G N P K V K A H G K K V L—T S F G
β Platypus ....... V H L S G G E K S A V T N L W G K V——N I N E——L G G E A L G R L L V V Y P W T Q R F F E A F G D L S S A G A V M G N P K V K A H G A K V L—T S F G
β Chicken ........ V H W T A E E K Q L I T G L W G K V——N V A E——C G A E A L A R L L I V Y P W T Q R F F A S F G N L S S P T A I L G N P M V R A H G K K V L—T S F G
β Shark .......... V H W S E V E L H E I T T T W K S I——D K H S——L G A K A L A R M F I V Y P W T T R Y F G N L K E F T A———————C S Y G V K E H A K K V T—G A L G
                                                        π    π π σ σ  σ σ   σ
                                                                    R
```

MYOGLOBIN (60 sequences; 27 invariant residues)

```
             1 2 3 4 5 6 7 8 9 10 11 12 13 14 15 16 17 18 19 20 21 22 23   24 25 26 27 28 29 30 31 32 33 34 35 36 37 38 39 40 41 42   43 44 45 46 47 48 49 50 51 52 53 54 55 56 57 58 59 60 61 62 63 64 65 66 67 68 69   70 71 72 73
Man ........ G—L S D G E W Q L V L N V W G K V E A D I P G——H G Q E V L I R L F K G H P E T L E K F D K F K H L K S E D E M K A S E D L K K H G A T V L—T A L G
Cow ........ G—L S D G E W Q A V L N A W G K V E A D V A G——H G Q E V L I R L F T G H P E T L E K F D K F K H L K T E A E M K A S E D L K K H G N T V L—T A L G
Sperm whale. V—L S E G E W Q L V L H V W A K V E A D V A G——H G Q D I L I R L F K S H P E T L E K F D R F K H L K T E A E M K A S E D L K K H G V T V L—T A L G
Platypus ... G—L S D G E W Q L V L K V W G K V E G D L P G——H G Q E V L I R L F K T H P E T L E K F D K F K G L K T E D E M K A S A D L K K H G G T V L—T A L G
Chicken .... G—L S D Q E W Q Q V L T I W G K V E A D I A G——H G H E V L M R L F H D H P E T L D R F D K F K G L K T E P D M K G S E D L K K H G Q T V L—T A L G
Shark ...... T E W E H V N K V W A V V E P D I P A——V G L A I L L R L F K E H K E T K D L F P K F K E I—P V Q Q L G N N E D L R K H G V T V L—R A L G
                                                       0  + + + 0 +  − 0 +  0
```

OTHER GLOBINS

```
Sea lamprey (Petromyzon) ....                                              0  + + + 0 0  0 0 0  0
   P I V D T G S V A P L S A A E K T K I R S A W A P V Y S N Y E T——S G V D I L V K F F T S T P A A Q E F F P K F K G L T T A D Q L K K S A D V R W H A E R I I—N A V N
Mollusc (Aplysia) ......... S—L S A A E A D L A G K S W A P V F A N K N A——N G A D F L V A L F E K F P D S A N F F A D F K G—K S V A D I K A S P X L R D V S S R I F—T R L N
Marine worm (Glycera) ... G—L S A A Q R Q V I A A T W K D I A G N D N G A G V G K D C L I K H L S A H P Q M A A V F—G F S G—A S D P A V———A D L———G A K V L—A Z I G
Midge larva (Chironomus) ..... L S A D Q I S T V Q A S F D K V K G D P———V G I L Y A——V F K A D P S I M A K F T Q F A G—K D L E S I K G T A P F E T H A N R I V—G F F S
Soybean leghemoglobin .. V A F T E K Q D A L V S S S F E A F K A N I P Q——Y S V V F Y T S I L E K A P A A K D L F S F L———A N G V D—P T N P K L T G H A E K L F—A L V R
Lupine leghemoglobin ... G V L T D V Q V A L V K S S F E E F N A N I P K——N T H R F F T L V L E I A P G A K D L F S F L K G—S S E V P—Q N N P D L Q A H A G K V F—K L T Y
```

Representative selection of amino acid sequences for the α and β hemoglobin families, myoglobin, and other monomeric globins. Sequences are displayed in the one-letter code of Figure 1.8 (B = Asp or Asn; Z = Glu or Gln). Light-color bars extending from Man through Platypus within one type of chain indicate positions that are invariant in all known mammals (not just those shown here) but are found to vary in at least some other vertebrates. Bars extending all the way down through shark indicate positions that are invariant in all known vertebrates for a given chain type. Darker color bars mark positions invariant in all known vertebrates and for all three hemoglobin and myoglobin chain types, or at two positions (CD1 and F8), for invertebrate globins as well.

The symbols π and σ in Table 3.1 mark the amino acid side chains that are involved in packing ($\alpha_1\beta_1$ and $\alpha_2\beta_2$) contacts and sliding ($\alpha_1\beta_2$ and $\alpha_2\beta_1$) contacts, respectively, between hemoglobin subunits. These regions tend to be strongly conserved, for obvious reasons: Mutations that radically change the character of these amino acids upset the operation of the hemoglobin molecule. The sliding-contact region occupies the center of the drawing in Figure 3.2a. The sliding contacts at the FG corner and beginning of the G helix are more strongly conserved than the packing contacts occurring later along the G and H helices

```
  E18 EF1              F1  F4    F8 FG1       G1    G5    G10         G17 GH1    H1          H10           H19  HC2
   :   :                :   :     :   :        :     :     :           :    :     :           :             :    :
68 69 70 71 72 73      76 77 78 79 80 81 82 83 84 85 86 87 88 89 90   91 92 93 94 95 96 97 98 99 100 102 104 106 108 110 112 114 116 118 120 122 124 126 128 130 132 134 136 138 140
N A V A H V D D ------- M P N A L S A L S D L H A H K --- L R V D P V N F K L L S H C L L V T L A A H L P A E F T P A V H A S L D K F L A S V S T V L T S K Y R
L A V G H V D D ------- M P N A L S A L S D L H A H K --- L R V D P V N F K L L S H C L L V T L A A H L P A E F T P A V H A S L D K F L A S V S T V L T S K Y R
K A V E H L D D ------- L P G A L S E L S D L H A H K --- L R V D P V N F K L L S H S L L V T L A S H L P S D F T P A V H A S L D K F L A N V S T V L T S K Y R
T A A G H F D D ------- M D S A L S A L S D L H A H K --- L R V D P V N F K L L A H C I L V V L A R H C P G E F T P S A H A A M D K F L S K V A T V L T S K Y R
N A I E H A D D ------- I S G A L S K L S D L H A H K --- L R V D P V N F K L L G Q C F L V V L V A H L P A E L A P K V H A S L D K F L C A V G T V L T A K Y R
D A V K S I D D ------- I G G A L S K L S E L H A Y I --- L R V D P V N F K L L S H C L L V T L A A R F P S D F T A E A H A A W D K F L S V V S S V L T E K Y R
D A V S K I D D ------- L V G G L A S L S E L H A S K --- L R V D P A N F K I L A N H I V V G I M F Y L P G D F P P E V H M S V D K F F Q N L A L A L S E K Y R
K A C D H L D D ------- L K T H L H K L A T F H G S E --- L K V D P A N F Q Y L S Y C L E V A L A V H L - T E F S P E T H C A L D K F L T N V C H E L S S R Y R
                                                          σ σ   σ σ σ σ σ     π         π       π π     π π   π π π     π π     π π           σ σ
                                                          T             R         R                                              R                      T
```

```
73 74 75 76 77 78 79 80      81 82 83 84 85 86 87 88 89 90 91 92 93 94 95   96 97 98 99 100 102 104 106 108 110 112 114 116 118 120 122 124 126 128 130 132 134 136 138 140 142 144 146
D G L N H L D N ----------- L K G T F A Q L S E L H C D K --- L H V D P E N F K L L G N V L V C V L A H H F G K E F T P Q V Q A A Y Q K V V A G V A N A L A H K Y H
D G L A H L D N ----------- L K G T F A T L S E L H C D K --- L H V D P E N F R L L G N V L V C V L A H H F G K E F T P P V Q A A Y Q K V V A G V A N A L A H K Y H
D G L A H L D N ----------- L K G T F S Q L S E L H C D K --- L H V D P E N F R L L G N V L V C V L A R N F G K E F T P Q M Q A A Y Q K V V A G V A N A L A H K Y H
D G M K H L D D ----------- L K G T F A A L S E L H C D K --- L H V D P E N F K L L G N V L V V V L A R N F G N E F T P V L Q A D F Q K V V A G V A N A L A H R Y H
E G L K Q L D D ----------- L K G A F A S L S E L H C D K --- L H V D P E N F R L L G N V L V V V L A R R F G S E F S P E L Q A S F Q K V V T G V A N A L A H R Y H
D A I K H L D D ----------- L K G T F A Q L S E L H C D K --- L H V D P E N F K L L G N V L V T V L A I H F G K E F T P E V Q A S W Q K M V T G V A S A L S S R Y H
D A I K N M D N ----------- L K P A F A K L S E L H C D K --- L H V D P E N F K L L G N V M V I I L A T H F G K E F T P E V Q A A W Q K L V S A V A I A L A H K Y H
D A L K N L D D ----------- L K G T F A K L S E L H C D K --- L H V D P E N F N R L G N V L V R H F S K D F S P E V Q A A W Q K L V S G V A H A L G H K Y H
D A V K N L D N ----------- I K N T F S Q L S E L H C D K --- L H V D P E N F R L L G D I L I I V L A A H F S K D F T P E C Q A A W Q K L V R V V A H A L A R K Y H
V A V T H L G D ----------- V K S Q F T D L S K K H A E E --- L H V D V E S F K L L A K C F V V E L G I L L K D K F A P Q T Q A I W E K Y F G V V V D A I S K E Y H
                                                             σ σ σ   σ σ   π σ     π       π     π π     π     π π π π   π π     π
                                                             T       R   R T                                   T                                           T T
```

```
74 75 76 77 78 79 80 81      82 83 84 85 86 87 88 89 90 91 92 93 94 95 96   97 98 99 100 102 104 106 108 110 112 114 116 118 120 122 124 126 128 130 132 134 136 138 140 142 144 146 148 150 152
G I L K K K G H ---------- H E A E I K P L A Q S H A T K --- H K I P V K Y L E F I S E C I I Q V L Q S K H P G D F G A D A Q G A M N K A L E L F R K D M A S N Y K E L G F Q G
G I L K K K G H ---------- H E A E V K H L A E S H A N K --- H K V P I K Y L E F I S D A I I H V L A K H P S N F A A D A Q G A M S K A L E L F R N D A A E K Y K V L G F H G
A I L K K K G H ---------- H E A E L K P L A Q S H A T K --- H K I P I K Y L E F I S E A I I H V L H S R H P G D F G A D A Q G A M N K A L E L F R K D I A A K Y K E L G Y Q G
N I L K K K G Q ---------- H E A E L K P L A Q S H A T K --- H K I S I K F L E Y I S E A I I H V L Q S K H S A D F G A D A Q A A M G K A L E L F R N D M A A K Y K E F G F Q G
A Q L K K K G H ---------- H E A D L K P L A Q T H A T K --- H K I P V K Y L E F I S E V I I K V I A E K H A A D F G A D S Q A A M K K A L E L F R D D M A S K Y K E F G F Q G
N I L K Q K G K ---------- H S T N V K E L A D T H I N K --- H K I P P K N F V L I T N I A V K V L T E M Y P S D M I G P M Q E S F S K V F T V I C S D L E T L Y K E A D F Q G
                                                            + 0 0   - 0 + -   0 0       +       0           + 0       0 0   0 0 0 +   0 0       0 0                       0 0
```

```
                                                            0 0 0 0 0 0   - 0 0     0         +     0 0             + 0     0 0                         0
D A V A S M D D T E --- K M S --- M K N L S G K H A K S --- F Q D P Q Y F K V L A A V I A D T V A A ----------- G D A G F E K L R M I C I L - L R S A Y
E F V N D A A N A G --- K M S A M L S Q F A K E H V G F G V G S A Q F E N V R S M F P G F V A S V A A ----------- P P A G A D A W T K L F G L I I D A L K A A G K
V A V S H L G D Z G --- K M V A Q M K A V G V R H K G Y G N K H I K G Q Y F E P L G A S L L S A M E H R I G G K M N A A A K D A W A A A Y A D I S G A L I S G L Q S
K I I G E L P N I E A D V N T F V --- A S K H P - R G V T H D Q L N N F R A G F V S Y M K A --- H T --- D F A G A E - A A W G A T L D T F F G M I F S K M
D S A G Q L K A - S G T V V A D A A L --- G S V H A Q K A V T --- N P - E F - V V K E A L L K T I K A A V G D K W S D E L S R A W E V A Y D E L A A A I K A K
E A A I Q L E V - N G A V A S D A T L K S L G S V H V S K G V V --- D A - H F P V V K E A I L K T I K E V V G D K W S E E L N T A W T I A Y D E L A I I I K K E M K D A A
```

Packing contacts between α_1 and β_1 subunits (or α_2 and β_2) are marked by π. Sliding contacts between α_1 and β_2 subunits (or α_2 and β_1) are marked by σ. T and R below these Greek letters indicate contacts only in the deoxy or the oxy configuration, respectively. Symbols +, 0, and − indicate increased, same, and decreased polarity, respectively, in myoglobin or in lamprey side chains, by comparison with the equivalent position in hemoglobin α and β chains where subunits come in contact. All sequences shown are from references 12 and 13, except for human ζ, which is from reference 14, and human ε, from reference 15. Note that the penultimate tyrosine, HC2 in hemoglobin, is H23(146) in the longer final H helix of myoglobin.

Figure 3.2(a) Color dots indicate the positions of invariant residues in mammalian hemoglobin sequences. There are 50 invariant positions in the 47 currently known mammalian α chain sequences, and 51 invariant positions in the 58 mammalian β family chains. Note that the α₁β₂ interface is almost totally conserved, as are the heme pockets. See Table 3.1, where mammalian invariants are shown by color bars: shorter bars for mammals only, and longer bars for invariants in mammals and other vertebrates.

(Table 3.1). This, again, is reasonable; moving parts are more easily disturbed by random changes than are static contact zones.

The symbols +, 0, and − below the myoglobin and above the lamprey sequences in Table 3.1 show whether those side chains that correspond to subunit contacts in hemoglobin are more polar (+), of similar polarity (0), or less polar (−) in myoglobin or lamprey than in the hemoglobin chains. Since these hemoglobin contact regions are in myoglobin exposed to the aqueous surroundings, one would expect the myoglobin side chains to be more polar, and this generally is true. (Lamprey will be discussed in Section 3.2.) Phe or Tyr at position C1 in hemoglobin α and β chains becomes His in myoglobin; Phe/Tyr C7 in hemoglobin becomes Lys or Arg in myoglobin; Leu FG3 in hemoglobin becomes His in myoglobin; and Val/Ile/Cys G14 in hemoglobin becomes Gln/His/Lys in myoglobin. This illustrates one way in which amino acid sequences can control the organization of multisubunit proteins. Certain regions on the surface of the individual hemoglobin subunits will favor aggregation because such aggregation buries nonpolar side chains, whereas myoglobin molecules fail to aggregate because the corresponding regions are polar. Both the

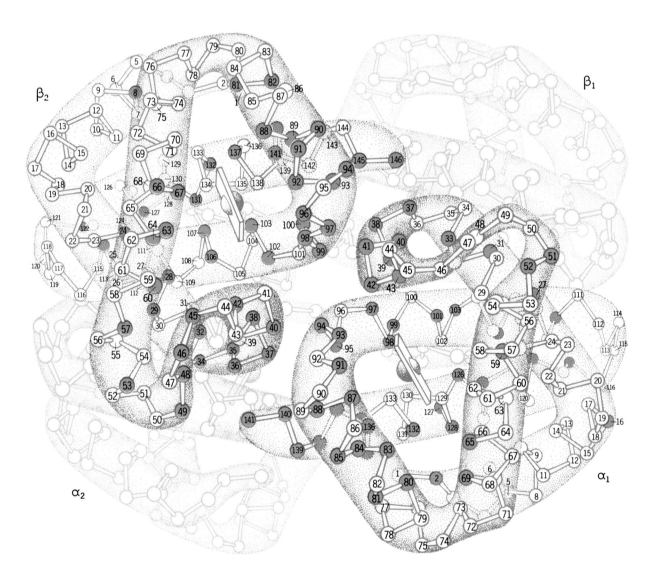

folding of each polypeptide chain and the aggregation of different chains are controlled by amino acid sequence.

Invariant positions for α and β chains of hemoglobin are shown by color dots in Figures 3.2(a) and (b) for mammals and for all vertebrates, respectively. Not surprisingly, these cluster around the centers of activity of the molecule: the heme crevice and the $\alpha_1\beta_2$ intersubunit contacts. In contrast, the outside of the molecule, far removed from these critical contacts, is more variable. In myoglobin (Figures 3.2(c) and (d)) the pattern is quite different: Invariant residues are widely scattered over the molecule, and there are more of them than in the hemoglobin chains. They probably reflect a need to stabilize the molecule as a whole, rather than specific working interfaces such as the C helix and the FG corner. The reason for the greater overall conservatism of myoglobin is less clear, but may arise from the fact that myoglobin sits unprotected in a milieu replete with enzymatic hazards in the cytoplasm of voluntary muscle cells, whereas hemoglobin finds a sheltered existence in virtually saturated solution within the erythrocytes.

Figure 3.2(b) In the same convention as Figure 3.2(a), invariant residues are shown for all currently known vertebrate sequences. In the α chains, 23 invariant positions are found among 60 species, and the β chains have 20 invariant positions among 66 species. These are indicated in Table 3.1 by the longer color bars extending from man to shark in each chain type.

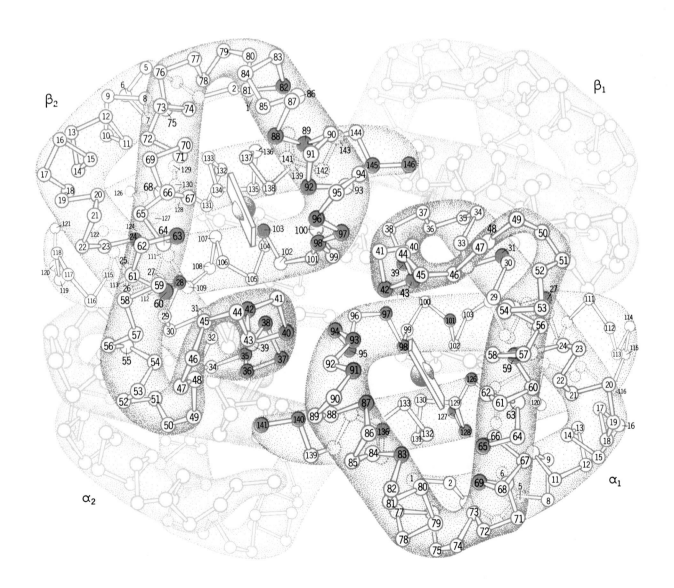

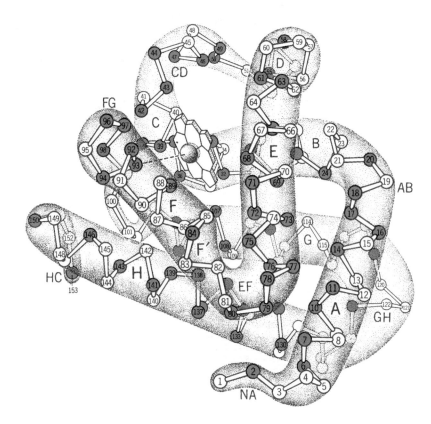

Figure 3.2(c) Color dots indicate the 71 invariant positions among 55 currently known mammalian myoglobin sequences. Note how the pattern differs from that in tetrameric hemoglobin in Figure 3.2(a). Invariant positions in myoglobin are widely scattered over the entire molecule, rather than being concentrated around the heme pocket, FG corner, and C helix. Nearly half the positions are invariant.

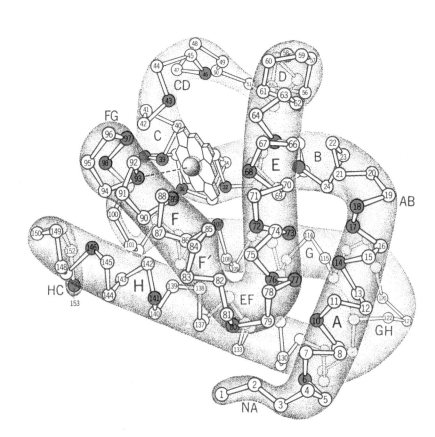

Figure 3.2(d) Positions of the 27 invariant residues in all 60 vertebrate myoglobin sequences. Note that the wide distribution of invariants is preserved in vertebrates, even though only 18% of the positions are unchanging. The sequences compared in preparing Figures 3.2(a–d) are identified in Appendix 3.2.

TABLE 3.2 HIGHLY CONSERVED RESIDUES IN VERTEBRATE HEMOGLOBIN
AND MYOGLOBIN[a]

I. Invariant in Table 2.3, also invariant in all known vertebrate sequences:

A. HYDROPHOBIC	B. POLAR OR AMBIVALENT
CD1 (phe)	C4 (thr)
F4 (leu)	F8 (his)
H23 or HC2 (tyr)	

The five invariant residues in Section I of Table 3.2 are shown as dark color bars in Table 3.1

II. Invariant in Table 2.3, but variable in other sequences:

A. HYDROPHOBIC	B. POLAR OR AMBIVALENT
NA2 (leu, trp, phe, tyr)	A14 (lys, his, ser, val[b])
A8 (val, leu, ile)	B6 (gly, ala)
A12 (trp, phe, leu, ser[b])	B12 (arg, ser)
A15 (val, leu, ile, ala, asn[b])	E5 (lys, arg, his, gln, leu[b])
B10 (leu, val)	E7 (his, gln)
C2 (pro, ala)	E8 (gly, ala)
CD4 (phe, trp, tyr, met, leu)	FG2 (lys, asp, glu, ile[b])
CD7 (leu, phe)	H10 (lys, ala)
E11 (val, ile)	H22 or HC1 (lys, arg, glu, asn, ala)
GH5 (phe, leu)	

[a]Underlining marks the predominant amino acid.
[b]A change in residue character has occurred.

3.2 SINGLE-CHAIN GLOBINS

The sequence comparisons in Table 3.1 also suggest that lamprey and invertebrate globins probably have the same chain folding as the vertebrates. Invertebrate globin genes tend to occur in multiple copies and to be polymorphic. That is, although the globin functions as a monomer, a given individual will have several genes producing similar but not identical chains. Sea lamprey (*Petromyzon*) has six globin genes, for example; bloodworm (*Glycera*) has at least four, and the midge (*Chironomus*) has more than ten. Only one example of each is given in Table 3.1; the others differ at a few amino acid positions. It is not clear why an invertebrate whose globin operates as a single chain should have several slightly different genes for that chain, but perhaps this represents a pool of genetic diversity from which the more highly organized globins of the vertebrates could evolve.

The identity of three-dimensional folding of several of these monomeric globins with vertebrate globin chains has been shown directly by x-ray crystal-structure analyses: the globin or erythrocruorin of the larva of the midge *Chironomus thummii* (A1–A4), hemoglobins of the sea lamprey *Petromyzon marinus* (A5, A6) and the marine bloodworm *Glycera dibranchiata* (A7, A8), and leghemoglobin from root nodules of the yellow lupine, *Lupinus luteus* (A9–A11). Stereo views of the chain folding for the first three of these are compared with those of the vertebrate globins in Figure 3.3. The pedigree of the globin gene can be traced at least to the divergence of various animal phyla in the late Precambrian, around 600–700 million years ago.

The occurrence of globins among invertebrates is quite irregular, and cannot be correlated in any simple way with classical phylogenetic trees (16). Some organisms that live in a plentiful oxygen supply may not produce a globin at all, whereas a closely related species that inhabits a more anoxic environment may have a globin that it uses as an oxygen-storage reservoir. Crustaceans inhabiting

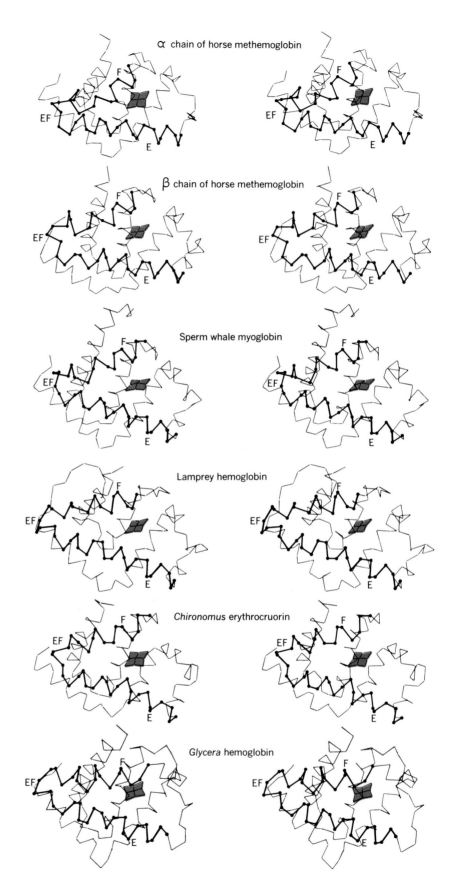

Figure 3.3 Polypeptide backbone chain folding in vertebrate and invertebrate globins. Each molecule is oriented with its F helix close to the viewer and the EF corner at the left. The heme is represented by a puckered colored square in the heme pocket. Each bend along a chain marks the position of an α carbon. (From reference A7.)

mud deposits that are kept relatively free of oxygen by the oxidation of rotting organic matter frequently possess more globin than their close relatives living in aerated water. Many insects such as the midge have a globin in their fast-growing larval stage, but lose it after metamorphosis in favor of the diffusion of gaseous oxygen through tracheal tubes. The water flea reacts to anoxia by synthesizing globin, but shuts down the synthesis as soon as it encounters a high oxygen concentration again. Three explanations can be proposed:

1. Invertebrates that possess a globin gene have received it from an outside source, and have retained it because it is useful to survival.

2. Globin genes have evolved repeatedly and independently in different invertebrate lines, from the gene for a different but related protein that they all possess.

3. All invertebrates began with a globin gene, but many have either lost it or turned it off by some kind of genetic control mechanism because they did not need it for oxygen storage or transport.

Hypothesis 1 is unlikely to be true, since lateral transfer of genetic information is not as easy in higher organisms as it is in bacteria. It cannot be absolutely excluded, however. Hypothesis 2 is more plausible, and cytochrome *a* has been suggested as the ancestral protein because it has the same type of heme group. But we do not have enough sequence information yet about cytochrome *a* to make a judgment. Hypothesis 3 perhaps is the most likely, especially in view of what has been said about organisms that can turn their globin genes on and off as the surrounding oxygen supply requires. The irregular occurrence of globins among invertebrates is more likely a matter of gene *expression* rather than gene *possession*.

Perhaps the most puzzling of all globins is leghemoglobin of the nitrogen-fixing root nodules of legumes. These nodules contain colonies of symbiotic bacteria, which actually contribute the nitrogen fixation process. Leghemoglobin is coded by a gene from the host plant, not the bacterium, although this might only mean that the gene was transferred from symbiont to host at some earlier time. In some cases the host plant needs a stimulus from the bacteria in its root nodules in order to commence making the leghemoglobin. A puzzling feature is that nitrogen fixation is a strictly anaerobic process: Free oxygen displaces sulfur from the nitrogenase enzyme and poisons it. Why would legumes want a globin in their root nodules? The answer may be that the globin is there as a scavenger to *remove* any traces of residual oxygen, thus preventing it from interfering with the nitrogen fixation process. If so, then this would be the only known case where the function of a globin was to eliminate oxygen rather than to supply it.

Shark and higher bony fish have the familiar tetrameric hemoglobin, with α and β chains. The more primitive lamprey employs only a single chain (even though it manufactures six slightly different variants of it), but behaves as if it were at an intermediate stage of development between monomers and tetramers. Lamprey deoxyglobin forms dimers, but the dimers dissociate when they bind oxygen:

$$Gl_2 + 2O_2 \rightleftarrows Gl \cdot O_2 + Gl \cdot O_2$$

Here Gl indicates globin. Hendrickson has found evidence from difference-map projections of lamprey globin in various states of ligation to suggest that when ligands bind to the heme in the crystal, slight shifts in chain conformation are induced in the C helix and the FG corner (17). These are just the $\alpha_1\beta_2$ and $\alpha_2\beta_1$ sliding contacts of tetrameric hemoglobin, seen in Figures 2.22 and 3.2. As has been mentioned, the $+$, 0, and $-$ above the lamprey sequence in Table 3.1 indicate an increase, no change, or decrease in polarity of side chains in going from vertebrate hemoglobin α and β to lamprey chains. Regions of sliding contact, marked in Table 3.1 by σ for the vertebrates, generally are of similar polarity in lamprey and vertebrates, whereas regions of packing contact ($\alpha_1\beta_1$ and $\alpha_2\beta_2$) in tetrameric hemoglobin, marked by π, generally are *more polar* in lamprey. This suggests that the sliding contacts of the vertebrate tetramer have their counterpart in the lamprey dimer, but that the packing contacts of the tetramer are exposed to the aqueous surroundings in lamprey. The deletion of nine residues of lamprey at the GH corner may also upset the packing contacts and make a tetramer impossible. The loss of the bond involving Asp G4 (which is Tyr in lamprey as well as in most myoglobins) may be enough to disrupt dimerization in the oxy state, which has intrinsically fewer subunit interactions than the deoxy state in vertebrates (See Table 2.4).

Hence a picture emerges, from the clues that have been given, of a lamprey globin that dimerizes in the deoxy state, using C helix and FG corner contacts analogous to the sliding contacts in vertebrate tetramers. When O_2 binds to the hemes, motion at the FG corners comparable to that in the switch regions in vertebrate tetramers pushes the dimers apart. Lacking the other two chains to furnish a flexible joint, they fall apart into monomers. When removal of oxygen allows the FG corners to shift back, then two chains can recombine into a dimer. If this line of reasoning is correct, then both the inability of lamprey globin to tetramerize, and its dimerization only in the deoxy state, are understandable at the molecular level. The other monomeric globins in Table 3.1 have deletions in the packing-contact regions (*Aplysia*, *Chironomus*) or sliding-contact regions (leghemoglobins), or increased polarity and altered charge distribution in contact zones (*Glycera*).

3.3   EVOLUTION OF THE GLOBIN FAMILY

The great similarity of amino acid sequences and three-dimensional folding in all of these globins makes it almost certain that their genes evolved by divergence from one ancestral globin gene. All of these proteins, therefore, make up one large evolutionarily related family. The differences between members of this family are shown in Table 3.3, which lists the number of amino acid changes in all pairwise comparisons of sequences. Such a *difference matrix* is one of the most useful tools in studying protein evolution.

In generating a difference matrix, those positions where one chain being compared has an amino acid but the other has a gap or deletion could be treated in two different ways. The position could simply be ignored, in which case one would be tallying the number of differences in those portions of chain that the two sequences had in common. These are designated as *common differences,* and appear above the diagonal in Table 3.3. They underestimate true evolutionary differences, since deletions themselves are evolutionary events. Alternatively, each deletion in one chain could be treated formally as a twenty-first kind of amino acid, when paired against a real amino acid in the other chain. This is the practice followed in the Dayhoff *Atlas* (12), and these figures, designated *all differences,* appear below the diagonal in Table 3.3. They overestimate evolutionary change, since the deletion of a 15-residue loop of chain by crossing over at the chromosomal level does not require as many separate events as 15

TABLE 3.3 DIFFERENCE MATRIX FOR GLOBIN SEQUENCES OF TABLE 3.1[a]

	Man α	Rhesus α	Cow α	Platypus α	Chicken α	Man ζ	Carp α	Shark α	Rhesus β	Man β	Man δ	Cow β	Cow "γ"	Man γ	Man ε	Platypus β	Chicken β	Shark β	Mb Man	Mb Cow	Mb Whale	Mb Platypus	Mb Chicken	Mb Shark	Sea lamprey	Mollusc	Glycera	Chironomus	Soybean	Lupine
α Man		4	17	39	35	61	68	79	75	75	76	78	82	80	83	81	81	91	103	101	103	101	100	103	82	106	104	98	108	117
α Rhesus	4		16	37	35	62	68	79	75	75	78	78	82	80	83	80	81	91	104	102	104	101	101	104	84	107	103	95	108	118
α Cow	17	16		44	38	60	65	75	75	76	78	78	80	79	83	76	80	92	102	101	102	100	100	101	85	108	100	92	108	117
α Platypus	39	37	44		47	66	74	80	73	73	74	72	78	78	76	77	79	92	98	99	101	97	98	104	89	109	104	96	107	111
α Chicken	35	35	38	47		69	72	83	83	85	87	87	85	84	84	85	87	93	109	106	108	104	107	105	92	110	109	99	109	118
ζ Man	61	62	60	66	69		70	90	85	87	85	87	85	82	83	82	79	99	103	99	101	102	102	97	84	108	100	101	104	114
α Carp	71	71	68	77	75	73		85	77	78	80	79	75	77	79	76	86	90	108	103	108	108	106	105	89	111	110	104	106	110
α Shark	88	88	84	89	92	99	95		93	92	92	92	89	85	91	86	92	89	110	111	113	111	112	107	105	110	106	103	112	116
β Rhesus	84	84	84	82	92	94	87	109		8	11	26	33	37	35	35	44	88	108	104	109	106	105	104	98	110	106	101	109	116
β Man	84	84	85	82	94	96	88	108	8		10	24	32	39	36	34	45	91	109	103	108	105	105	103	97	112	106	98	109	117
δ Man	85	87	87	83	96	94	90	108	11	10		26	33	41	40	38	45	91	108	104	109	106	106	101	97	108	106	100	109	116
β Cow	86	86	86	80	95	95	88	107	27	25	27		23	39	41	40	54	91	112	107	112	109	110	104	94	115	106	105	110	116
"γ" Cow	90	90	88	86	93	93	84	104	34	33	34	23		39	39	38	52	93	110	106	110	109	109	100	95	110	109	102	106	110
γ Man	89	89	88	87	93	91	87	101	37	39	41	40	40		30	40	44	86	109	108	112	110	107	104	95	111	105	105	107	113
ε Man	92	92	92	85	93	92	89	107	35	36	40	42	40	30		37	37	91	111	107	110	110	108	108	96	109	110	103	105	113
β Platypus	90	89	85	86	94	91	86	102	35	34	38	41	39	40	37		42	90	101	101	106	102	101	106	96	101	104	101	108	115
β Chicken	90	90	89	88	96	91	88	108	44	45	45	55	53	44	37	42		86	107	103	107	105	105	105	96	101	106	101	108	115
β Shark	95	95	96	96	97	103	95	100	93	96	96	97	99	91	96	95	91		110	110	109	111	109	107	94	107	105	102	111	116
Mb Man	115	116	114	110	121	115	121	129	117	118	117	120	118	118	120	110	116	124		29	25	25	35	83	104	110	106	103	118	118
Mb Cow	113	114	113	111	118	117	116	130	113	112	113	115	114	117	116	110	112	124	29		30	36	45	87	101	110	111	103	119	122
Mb Whale	115	116	114	113	120	113	121	132	118	117	118	120	118	121	119	115	116	123	25	30		31	43	85	102	106	108	103	113	120
Mb Platypus	113	113	112	109	116	114	121	130	115	114	115	117	117	119	119	111	114	125	25	36	31		37	85	102	108	108	98	116	117
Mb Chicken	112	113	112	110	119	114	119	131	114	114	115	118	117	116	117	110	114	123	35	45	43	37		85	101	108	109	101	114	114
Mb Shark	120	121	118	121	122	114	123	131	118	117	115	117	113	118	122	120	119	126	88	92	90	90	90		100	108	114	106	113	116
Sea lamprey	113	115	116	120	123	115	121	127	124	123	123	121	122	121	122	122	122	125	135	132	133	133	132	136		95	97	100	105	112
Mollusc	124	125	126	127	128	126	130	133	125	127	123	129	124	126	124	124	116	127	128	128	124	126	126	131	114		106	101	108	112
Glycera	124	123	120	124	129	120	129	133	125	125	125	124	127	124	129	123	125	127	126	131	128	128	129	139	132	122		98	108	112
Chironomus	131	128	125	129	132	134	138	141	131	128	130	134	131	135	133	131	131	137	136	136	136	131	134	142	138	124	129		104	107
Soybean	131	131	131	130	132	127	132	144	131	131	131	133	129	129	127	129	130	136	145	146	140	143	141	145	143	131	135	128		62
Lupine	137	138	137	131	138	134	131	143	133	134	133	134	128	130	130	130	132	136	134	138	136	133	130	137	147	130	132	134	73	

[a]Above the diagonal, positions with deletions in either chain are not included (*common differences*); below the diagonal, a deletion in one chain is counted as a difference (*all differences*).

individual amino acid alterations by point mutation. Both methods give comparable results for chains as similar as these globins are. However, with more extensive insertions and deletions as in the bacterial cytochromes *c*, the two methods begin to reveal different information. In the discussion that follows, we shall use the *all-differences* figures below the diagonal of the table.

The most striking observation from Table 3.3 is that the hemoglobins and myoglobins do make up quite separate subfamilies, with the differences within one subfamily (fewer than 110 changes) being smaller than those between myoglobin and hemoglobin sequences (110–132 changes). Furthermore, the invertebrate globins differ more from one another and from all the vertebrate chains (113–146 changes) than the vertebrate myoglobins differ from either hemoglobin chain. Starting from the common invertebrate heritage of a cluster of genes manufacturing a single-chain globin, the vertebrates apparently developed two specialized genes: one for an oxygen-storing myoglobin and the other for an oxygen-carrying hemoglobin monomer. The hemoglobin gene or genes later specialized into genes for distinct α and β chains, leading to the tetramer that we know today.

Within the α or β hemoglobin chains a strong correlation exists between the number of changes between species, and the distance apart of those species on the traditional phylogenetic tree. The α chains of man and rhesus monkey differ by only 4 positions out of 141, cow and primates differ by 16 or 17, birds (chicken) and mammals by 35–47, bony fish (carp) and land vertebrates by 68–77, and cartilaginous fish (shark) and higher vertebrates by 84–99 residues. The human ζ gene appears to have split off from the α gene at some time before the reptilian ancestors of mammals and birds diverged. The numbers within the α-family box at the upper left corner of Table 3.3 suggest the phylogenetic tree shown in Figure 3.4. The only apparent anomaly is that the α hemoglobin sequence of platypus, a primitive monotreme mammal, seems more different from both chicken and the placental mammals than might have been expected from classical evolutionary biology.

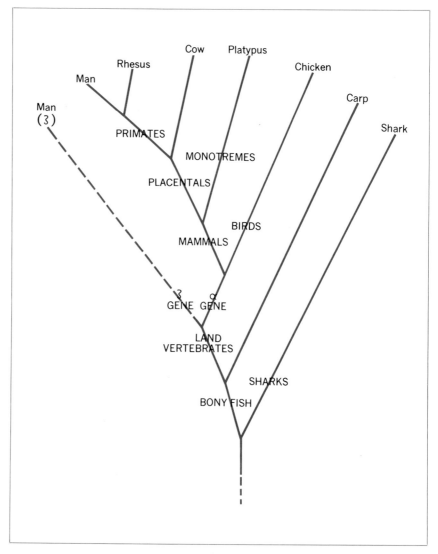

Figure 3.4 Schematic family tree of globin-containing vertebrates. The same tree is obtained by comparing sequences of myoglobin, or the α or β chains of hemoglobin, if one uses the general principle that closely similar sequences imply closely related species, and quite different sequences imply distantly related species. This tree, for the α chains, also shows the point at which α and ζ genes duplicated and went their separate ways.

TABLE 3.4 DIFFERENCE MATRIX FOR β, γ, AND δ CHAINS[a,b]

		Rhesus β	Man β	Man δ	Cow β	Cow "γ"	Man γ	Man ε	Platypus β	Chicken β	Shark β
β	Rhesus		7.7	10.8	28.9	32.7	37.3	35.9	36.4	44.0	94.3
β	Man	8		10.7	28.8	32.6	37.2	35.8	36.3	43.9	94.2
δ	Man	11	10		30.5	34.3	38.9	37.5	38.0	45.6	95.9
β	Cow	27	25	27		24.0	39.6	38.2	38.7	46.3	96.6
"γ"	Cow	34	33	34	23		43.4	42.0	42.5	50.1	100.4
γ	Man	37	39	41	40	40		29.4	37.1	44.7	95.0
ε	Man	35	36	40	42	40	30		35.7	43.3	93.6
β	Platypus	35	34	38	41	39	40	37		43.8	94.1
β	Chicken	44	45	45	55	53	44	37	42		92.1
β	Shark	93	96	96	97	99	91	96	95	91	

[a] At upper right are calculated values based on the tree shown in Figure 3.9; at lower left, observed values, all differences.
[b] rms discrepancy = 2.5.

The β chains tell the same story, except that the platypus anomaly is resolved. They provide independent confirmation of the phylogenetic tree of Figure 3.4, and all the accumulated evidence of classical biology tells us that this tree is correct. In globins as in other proteins a general principle seems to be valid: *The more distantly related two species are, the more dissimilar the sequences of shared proteins will be.* This implies that the genes for distantly related species, having separated a longer time in the past, have had more time in which to accumulate random but acceptable base mutations. Some of these mutations may be acceptable because the resulting protein sequence actually is an improvement, making the protein function better. This is *positive* selection. Others may only have been allowed because they are harmless, having little effect on protein function. These are termed *neutral* mutations. Those mutations that led to an inferior protein, in contrast, would have been weeded out by natural selection, and would not be seen in the genetic record. So far this is only a qualitative principle, not necessarily implying that the number of differences need be proportional to the time elapsed since gene separation. The *order* of events in the tree is determined by the difference matrix, but not necessarily a linear time coordinate. This is sometimes called the "rubber-branched tree" model, since the lengths of individual branches are uncertain, although their connections are not.

If this principle is valid, then one should be able to use the data in Table 3.3 to decide the order in which the genes for the α, β, γ, δ, ε, and ζ hemoglobin chains diverged, relative to the divergence of species. The most obvious fact is that the α and β families themselves generally are more different than are any of the members of either family. Their differences are comparable with the differences between shark and the higher vertebrates within each α or β family, suggesting that the differentiation between α and β genes was taking place at about the same time as the separation of the cartilaginous and bony fish, or approximately 450–500 million years ago (18).

The multiplicity of β, γ, δ, and ε chains within the β family in Table 3.3 at first seems confusing, but the addition of ruled boxes as in the lower left half of Table 3.4 simplifies matters somewhat. Of all the sequences compared, the β

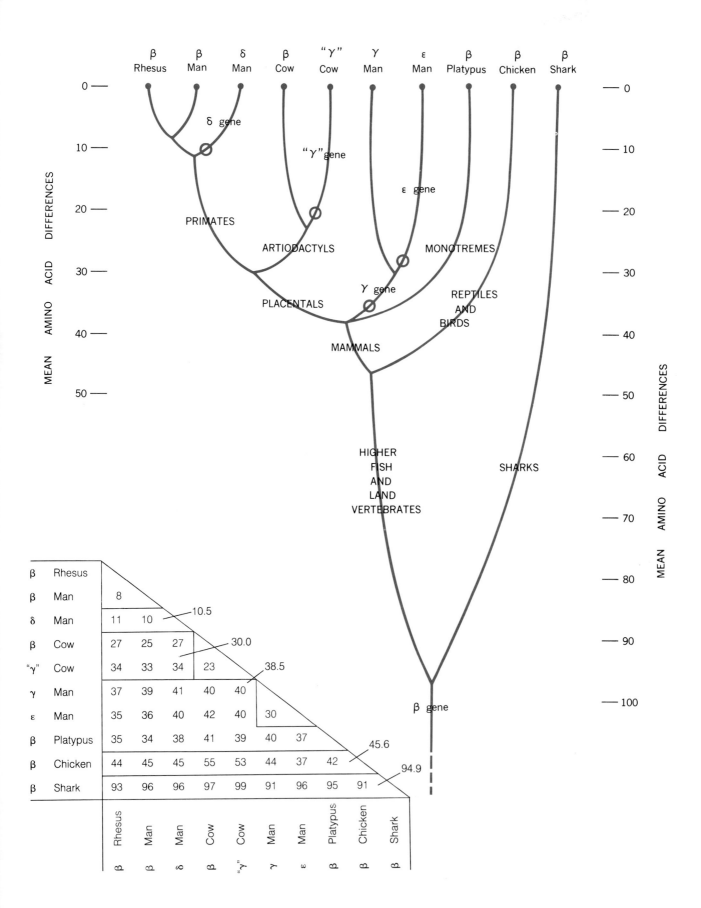

chains of man and rhesus monkey are most closely related (8 differences), followed by the δ chain of man (10–11 changes). (Rhesus monkey also has a δ chain, not included in this particular selection of sequences.) The β and γ chains of cow form their own subgroup (23 differences), and all five of these mammalian chains are more closely related to one another (25–34 differences) than to any of the remaining five sequences (34 or more changes). Human γ and ε chains form another subgroup with 30 differences. The mammals as a whole are separated from birds (chicken) by 37–55 differences, and all of these land vertebrates differ from shark by twice as much, 91–99 changes. All of these relationships are depicted in the tree shown in Figure 3.5. This tree is semi-quantitative, in the sense that the vertical distance down from the top to any branch point has been made proportional to the *average* number of differences between sequences on the two sides of the branch point. For example, the junction between primates and artiodactyls has been placed at 30.0 on the vertical scale because this is the average of the six differences between human β and δ and rhesus β on one side, and bovine β and γ on the other.

This tree suggests that the γ chain found in human fetal hemoglobin evolved by a doubling of the β gene during the same period in which the mammals were diverging from their egg-laying reptilian ancestors. Classical paleontology would place this in the early Cretaceous, approximately 120 million years ago (18). The tree also suggests that the embryonic human ε chain was a somewhat later offshoot of the γ gene, not the β. The γ chain of bovine fetal hemoglobin is seen from Figure 3.5 to have been a later independent development, since it is more like the bovine β chain than human γ. It should not properly be termed a γ chain at all, if that designation is reserved for descendants of the gene that produces the human fetal chain. For this reason, the bovine chain will hereafter be termed either fetal or "γ." Finally, the β gene in primates separated into β and δ genes at some time prior to the divergence of the ancestors of rhesus monkeys and the great apes.

Everything that has been said so far about the evolution of the globins from a common single-chain oxygen-binding ancestor is summarized in the composite tree of Figure 3.6. Divergences of species are indicated by simple tree branching, and points of gene duplication by numbered circles. The earliest of these gene divergences is the hemoglobin/myoglobin split at the bottom. Myoglobin undergoes no further diversification, but the hemoglobin gene differentiates into α and β during the evolution of fish. The α in turn subdivides into α and ζ somewhere in the reptilian line. On the β branch of the tree, β differentiates into adult β and fetal γ during the rise of mammals. The γ gene itself later produces both γ and ε, and on the other branch, cattle develop their own fetal chain whereas primates generate a δ. Note that after a gene duplication, *each* gene thereafter builds its own phylogenetic tree of subsequent species diversification. This is the main reason for restricting discussion here to a carefully selected group of sequences in Table 3.1. If all of the 186 vertebrate sequences were used, the simultaneous presentation of gene diversification and species differentiation in one tree would become so complex as to be unintelligible.

← **Figure 3.5** Semi-quantitative phylogenetic tree of β, γ, δ, and ε hemoglobin sequences. The distance down to each branch point is proportional to the average number of differences between all pairwise comparisons of sequences on the two sides of the branch. ◯ = gene duplication and appearance of a new gene. The portion of the difference matrix used in constructing this tree is also shown, with the averages used to position branch points indicated.

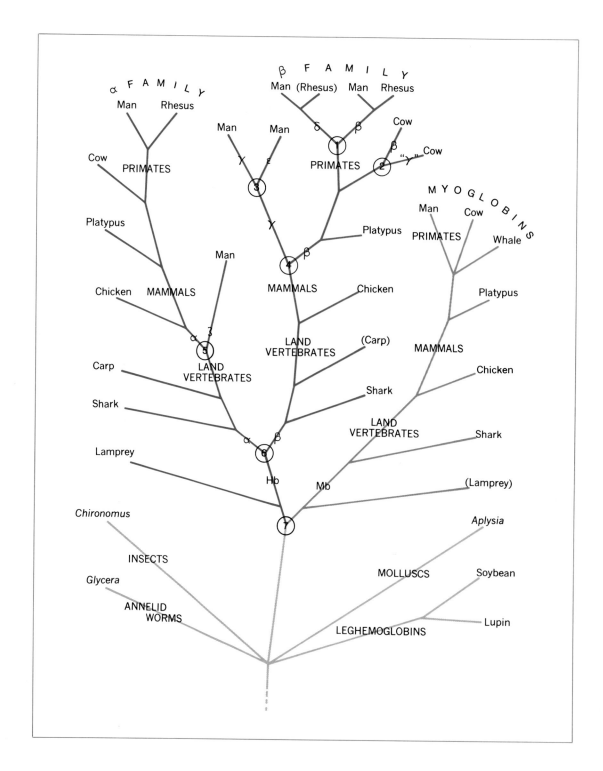

Figure 3.6 Composite tree of the globin family. This tree shows phylogenetic relationships among all of the species listed in Table 3.1. Branch points with numbered circles represent gene duplications, and simple unmarked branches are species divergences. Sequences of species in parentheses are not given in Table 3.1, but the species are included here for completeness. A myoglobin has been found in lamprey heart, but its sequence is not yet known. The separation of shark from bony fish is very close to the α/β gene duplication, point 6. The separation of lamprey from jawed fish is close to the hemoglobin/myoglobin split, point 7.

3.4 GLOBIN GENE STRUCTURE

All of the foregoing is consistent with what we know about the globins. Hemoglobin A, with composition $\alpha_2\beta_2$, makes up 97.5% of adult primate hemoglobin. Hemoglobin A_2, of composition $\alpha_2\delta_2$, is a minor component of uncertain function seen only in primates. Fetal hemoglobins, $\alpha_2\gamma_2$, with DPG insensitivity, are encountered only in mammals, and appear to have evolved independently in primates and in artiodactyls. Humans have three earlier embryonic hemoglobins using ζ (α-like) and ε (β-like) chains: Gower-1 of composition $\zeta_2\varepsilon_2$, Gower-2 or $\alpha_2\varepsilon_2$, and sometimes Portland or $\zeta_2\gamma_2$ (16, 19, 20). Humans actually have two γ genes adjacent on the same chromosome. One produces the sequence given in Table 3.1, and the other differs only by an alanine instead of glycine at position 136(H14). These are designated as the $^G\gamma$ and $^A\gamma$ genes, respectively.

The α and β families of hemoglobin genes are found on separate chromosomes in man, and the development of cloning methods has made it possible to map these regions of DNA, to locate the individual genes, and to determine the base sequences of segments thousands of bases long (20–22). The structures of the regions of DNA that contain the α and β families of genes are shown in Figure 3.7a. The 5′-to-3′ direction of each DNA chain is from left to right, but bases are numbered in thousands from right to left at the top of the figure. On human chromosome 16, which contains the α family, two widely spaced ζ genes come first, followed by a defective α-like "pseudogene," $\psi_{\alpha 1}$, that does not code for a protein chain, and finally two α genes labeled α_2 and α_1. The last four of these five genes are evenly spaced, approximately every 4000 bases along the chromosome. On human chromosome 11, an ε gene is followed after a long interval by the two $^G\gamma$ and $^A\gamma$ genes, another defective pseudogene, $\psi_{\beta 1}$, and then by the δ and β genes. It is interesting, and possibly important in gene regulation, that the order of genes from 5′ to 3′ along each chromosome is exactly the order in which the globin chains are needed during development from embryo to fetus to adult, and that in each case the adult chains are separated from the earlier genes by a pseudogene that looks like a defective version of the adult

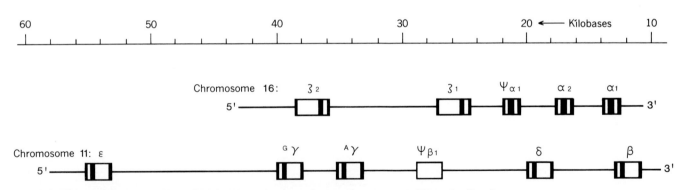

Figure 3.7(a) Arrangement of hemoglobin genes along two human chromosomes. The α family of genes lies along chromosome 16, and the β family is on chromosome 11. Rectangular boxes are the transcribed genes, and thin horizontal lines are the intervening untranscribed spacer DNA. *Exons,* destined for ultimate translation into amino acid sequences (see chapter-opening illustration), are represented by vertical black bands across the boxes, and *intron* sequences that are edited out from the messenger RNA are in white. $\psi_{\alpha 1}$ and $\psi_{\beta 1}$ are defective or pseudogenes, with sequence resemblances to true genes although they are not translated into protein chains. The exon–intron structure of $\psi_{\beta 1}$ is not known. The scale above gives DNA lengths in kilobases, measured from the right or 3′ end. This is a concrete example of the gene duplication sketched in Figure 3.1.

form. (This 5′-to-3′ order of genes is not found in all vertebrates, however. In chicken, two embryonic β genes flank the hatching and adult genes [23].) The actual base sequence of the human beta gene is shown in Figure 3.7b. With the help of the genetic code in Figure 3.10, you can verify that the base regions marked by color as *exons* do in fact correspond to the true human beta chain amino acid sequence.

The relative amounts of the various chains produced are plotted in Figure 3.8 against the time of pre- and postnatal development (24). The initial ζ and ε embryonic chains synthesized after conception are gradually replaced by α and γ chains during the first 8 weeks, and the original Gower-1 hemoglobin is replaced first by Gower-2 and Portland, and finally by hemoglobin F. Synthesis of β chain, minor at first, begins to accelerate around the thirty-fourth week of pregnancy. Within 3 weeks after birth, β and γ chains are in equal competition. At 6 months after birth, the adult $\alpha_2\beta_2$ form has essentially taken over, along with the minor $\alpha_2\delta_2$ component. Two pathological types of hemoglobin tetramer are known in humans: In α-thalassemia, a disease in which α-chain production is decreased or even eliminated, the excess γ and β chains can form tetramers of their own—hemoglobin Bart's (γ_4), or hemoglobin H (β_4). Both Bart's and H can bind oxygen, but do not display a Bohr effect or heme–heme cooperativity in O_2 binding.

Each of the globin genes in Figure 3.7 is separated from others by long base sequences that never are read out as messenger RNA (mRNA). These *flanking sequences* do however appear to be important in gene control and in the genetic recombination or scrambling that is one source of evolutionary diversity (20). Each globin gene also has within it two base sequences that are transcribed into mRNA, but then are edited out before the mRNA is used to direct protein synthesis at the ribosomes. These intervening sequences, called *introns*, are represented by gray bands across the genes in Figure 3.7. They separate three *exons*, which are regions of DNA that are destined to be translated into amino acid sequences. The exon-coded domains of hemoglobin are diagrammed in the chapter-opening illustration. In the α family of genes, these exons are 93, 204, and 126 bases long, respectively, and code for amino acid residues 1–31, 32–99, and 100–141. The two introns in the α genes are 127 and 134 bases long, and in

Figure 3.7(b) Nucleic acid sequence of the human β hemoglobin gene. Bases C, G, T, and A are listed from the 5′ end (position No. 1) to the 3′ end (No. 2052). Exons are colored, and introns have grey overprinting. Exon 1 begins with base No. 157, GTG = Val NA1, and ends at No. 246 to complete codon AGG = Arg B12. Exon 2 begins at No. 377, CTG = Leu B13 and ends with No. 598, AGG = Arg G6. The final exon 3 begins with base No. 1449, CTC = Leu G7, and ends at No. 1574 with CAC = His HC3. From the Nucleic Acid Database, Reference 12.

```
            10          20          30          40          50          60          70          80          90         100
   1 CCCTGTGGAG  CCACACCCTA  GGGTTGGCCA  ATCTACTCCC  AGGAGCAGGG  AGGGCAGGAG  CCAGGGCTGG  GCATAAAAGT  CAGGGCAGAG  CCATCTATTG
 101 CTTACATTTG  CTTCTGACAC  AACTGTGTTC  ACTAGCAACC  TCAAACAGAC  ACCATGGTGC  ACCTGACTCC  TGAGGAGAAG  TCTGCCGTTA  CTGCCCTGTG  EXON 1
 201 GGGCAAGGTG  AACGTGGATG  AAGTTGGTGG  TGAGGCCCTG  GGCAGGTTGG  TATCAAGGTT  ACAAGACAGG  TTTAAGGAGA  CCAATAGAAA  CTGGGCATGT
 301 GGAGACAGAG  AAGACTCTTG  GGTTTCTGAT  AGGCACTGAC  TCTCTCTGCC  TATTGGTCTA  TTTTCCCACC  CTTAGGCTGC  TGGTGGTCTA  CCCTTGGACC  EXON 2
 401 CAGAGGTTCT  TTGAGTCCTT  TGGGGATCTG  TCCACTCCTG  ATGCTGTTAT  GGGCAACCCT  AAGGTGAAGG  CTCATGGCAA  GAAAGTGCTC  GGTGCCTTTA
```

```
            10          20          30          40          50          60          70          80          90         100
 501 GTGATGGCCT  GGCTCACCTG  GACAACCTCA  AGGGCACCTT  TGCCACACTG  AGTGAGCTGC  ACTGTGACAA  GCTGCACGTG  GATCCTGAGA  ACTTCAGGGT
 601 GAGTCTATGG  GACCCTTGAT  GTTTTCTTTC  CCCTTCTTTT  CTATGGTTAA  GTTCATGTCA  TAGGAAGGGG  AGAAGTAACA  GGGTACAGTT  TAGAATGGGA
 701 AACAGACGAA  TGATTGCATC  AGTGTGGAAG  TCTCAGGATC  GTTTTAGTTT  CTTTTATTTG  CTGTTCATAA  CAATTGTTTT  CTTTTGTTTA  ATTCTTGCTT
 801 TCTTTTTTTT  TCTTCTCCGC  AATTTTTACT  ATTATACTTA  ATGCCTTAAC  ATTGTGTATA  ACAAAAGGAA  ATATCTCTGA  GATACATTAA  GTAACTTAAA
 901 AAAAAACTTT  ACACAGTCTG  CCTAGTACAT  TACTATTTGG  AATATATGTG  TGCTTATTTG  CATATTCATA  ATCTCCCTAC  TTTATTTTCT  TTTATTTTTA
```

```
            10          20          30          40          50          60          70          80          90         100
1001 ATTGATACAT  AATCATTATA  CATATTTATG  GGTTAAAGTG  TAATGTTTTA  ATATGTGTAC  ACATATTGAC  CAAATCAGGG  TAATTTTGCA  TTTGTAATTT
1101 TAAAAAATGC  TTTCTTCTTT  TAATATACTT  TTTTGTTTAT  CTTATTTCTA  ATACTTTCCC  TAATCTCTTT  CTTTCAGGGC  AATAATGATA  CAATGTATCA
1201 TGCCTCTTTG  CACCATTCTA  AAGAATAACA  GTGATAATTT  CTGGGTTAAG  GCAATAGCAA  TATTTCTGCA  TATAAATATT  TCTGCATATA  AATTGTAACT
1301 GATGTAAGAG  GTTTCATATT  GCTAATAGCA  GCTACAATCC  AGCTACCATT  CTGCTTTTAT  TTTATGGTTG  GGATAAGGCT  GGATTATTCT  GAGTCCAAGC
1401 TAGGCCCTTT  TGCTAATCAT  GTTCATACCT  CTTATCTTCC  TCCCACAGCT  CCTGGGCAAC  GTGCTGGTCT  GTGTGCTGGC  CCATCACTTT  GGCAAAGAAT  EXON 3
```

```
            10          20          30          40          50          60          70          80          90         100
1501 TCACCCCACC  AGTGCAGGCT  GCCTATCAGA  AAGTGGTGGC  TGGTGTGGCT  AATGCCCTGG  CCCACAAGTA  TCACTAAGCT  CGCTTTCTTG  CTGTCCAATT
1601 TCTATTAAAG  GTTCCTTTGT  TCCCTAAGTC  CAACTACTAA  ACTGGGGGAT  ATTATGAAGG  GCCTTGAGCA  TCTGGATTCT  GCCTAATAAA  AAACATTTAT
1701 TTTCATTGCA  ATGATGTATT  TAAATTATTT  CTGAATATTT  TACTAAAAAG  GGAATGTGGG  AGGTCAGTGC  ATTTAAAACA  TAAAGAAATG  ATGAGCTGTT
1801 CAAACCTTGG  GAAAATACAC  TATATCTTAA  ACTCCATGAA  AGAAGGTGAG  GCTGCAACCA  GCTAATGCAC  ATTGGCAACA  GCCCCTGATG  CCTATGCCTT
1901 ATTCATCCCT  CAGAAAAGGA  TTCTTGTAGA  GGCTTGATTT  GCAGGTTAAA  GTTTTGCTAT  GCTGTATTTT  ACATTACTTA  TTGTTTTAGC  TGTCCTCATG
```

```
            10          20          30          40          50          60          70          80          90         100
2001 AATGTCTTTT  CACTACCCAT  TTGCTTATCC  TGCATCTCTC  TCAGCCTTGA  CT
```

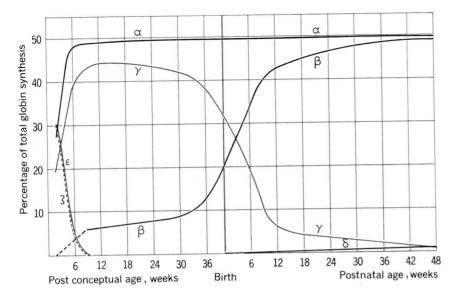

Figure 3.8 Relative amounts of α, β, γ, δ, ε, and ζ chains at different times in the development of the human embryo, fetus, and infant. The ζ chain is supplanted by the α early in the prenatal period. The ε chain is replaced by the γ at about the same time, and γ is replaced by β (and δ) shortly after birth. (From Reference 23.)

the ζ genes they are 1262 and 355 bases in length. On the other chromosome, all of the β family of genes have three exons coding for amino acid residues 1–30, 31–104, and 105–146. The first intron is 122–130 bases long, and the second is considerably longer, 850–914 bases. In both α and β genes the intron breaks occur after the codons for amino acid residues B12 and G6.

This pattern of exons and introns in the α and β families of human genes is quite old. Introns are found at exactly the same positions in the α and β genes of mouse, the β genes of rabbit, and the α and β genes of the South American toad *Xenopus laevis* (20, 25). The exon–intron–exon–intron–exon structure that we see today apparently developed prior to the split of α and β genes around 500 million years ago. Soybean leghemoglobin (26) has this same pattern, but with a third intron between the codons for Leu 68 and Val 69, or roughly after position E14. It would be interesting to see whether myoglobin genes also have the same internal structure, and whether they also have the extra leghemoglobin intron.

The role of introns is unknown. They tend to be under weaker selection pressure than the exons, as might seem reasonable since they do not code for amino acids in the final protein. Variation in base sequence has been observed in the $^G\gamma$, $^A\gamma$, δ, and β genes in a sample of 60 human individuals (27), but this variation is confined exclusively to the introns, meaning that the actual protein sequences are unchanged. The breaks between exons correspond roughly to natural structural domains within the folded globin subunits. (See chapter opening illustration.) Exon 1 corresponds to helices A and B; exon 2 builds the heme pocket and the $\alpha_1\beta_2$ sliding contacts from helix C to the middle of helix G; and exon 3 completes the last two helices including the $\alpha_1\beta_1$ packing contacts. It has been suggested that these exons represent a kind of modular construction scheme by which a functional protein might be developed from independent structural domains (28). If so, then this exon–intron arrangement could be important in gene evolution. The introns also seem to be necessary for the proper posttranscriptional processing of mRNA; one nonfunctional pseudogene in mouse has both introns neatly trimmed out, leaving a complete and uninterrupted exon sequence that nevertheless is useless in making β chains. The four exons in soybean leghemoglobin code for protein domains of similar length: 32, 36, 35, and 39 amino acids. As the opening figure of this chapter shows, these are the A helix and half of the B, the B-C-D-E bend to the middle of the E helix, the E and

F helices with the beginning of the G, and the G and H helices. These all are similar U- or V-shaped bends with α-helical arms, and this modular construction may possibly reflect the early evolution of the globin gene itself.

Figure 3.7 suggests that globin genes tend to come in pairs: ζ_2 and ζ_1, α_2 and α_1, $^G\gamma$ and $^A\gamma$, and perhaps even δ and β. The two ζ genes appear to have almost identical exon sequences so far as they are known, but ζ_1 may have a nonsense mutation that makes it really a pseudogene. The polypeptide products of $^G\gamma$ and $^A\gamma$ differ by a single amino acid, and those from the two α chains are identical as far as is known. It has been suggested that the γ genes and the α genes "talk to" their respective partners; that is, genetic recombination operates constantly to keep the sequences at the two γ or α loci effectively identical (29, 30). If such a mechanism ever existed for the δ and β genes, it has broken down in the primates, allowing the two genes to go their separate ways. For reasons that are not clearly understood, the nucleated bone marrow cells that are the precursors of mature erythrocytes have only one-tenth as much δ mRNA precursor as β, and mature red blood cells have no δ-chain messenger at all. The δ gene appears to be a defective or "spoiled" β gene, on its way to becoming only a pseudogene. Its failure is one of regulation at the messenger level, rather than one of functioning of the completed hemoglobin A_2 molecule, which apparently behaves normally.

3.5 PHYLOGENETIC TREES AND EVOLUTIONARY RATES

The composite tree in Figure 3.6 is purely schematic. Although it is topologically correct in the attachments of its branches, the distances along branches have no meaning, in terms of either evolutionary time or degree of sequence difference. The tree in Figure 3.5 is more quantitative, in that its branch points are positioned according to the average difference between sequences on opposite sides of the branch. One can go still further, and construct a tree with branches of variable length such that the distance down from each individual species to a branch point and back up to another species will match as closely as possible the observed difference between sequences. Such a tree is shown in Figure 3.9. If the various vertical distances between present-day species and branch points, or between branch points themselves, are defined by the variables a through p, then equations can be set up using the observed differences below the diagonal in Table 3.4.

$$a + b = 8 \quad \text{(the number of differences between human and rhesus β)}$$
$$a + c + d = 11 \quad \text{(rhesus β vs. human δ)}$$
$$b + c + d = 10 \quad \text{(human β vs. δ)}$$
$$g + h = 23 \quad \text{(cow β vs. "γ")}$$
$$a + c + e + f + g = 27 \quad \text{(β of rhesus vs. cow)}$$
$$\ldots \ldots \text{etc.}$$

One equation will result for every pairwise sequence comparison, or every number below the diagonal in Table 3.4, 45 in all. But there are only 16 branch lengths or variables to be determined, a through p. Hence the problem is overdetermined, and only an approximate best fit can be found. Furthermore, the attachment point of the ancestral stem (x in Figure 3.9) is not defined by the data in Table 3.4. Only the sum of the two bottommost branches, p, can be found, not their individual values. Various computer methods exist for obtaining the best

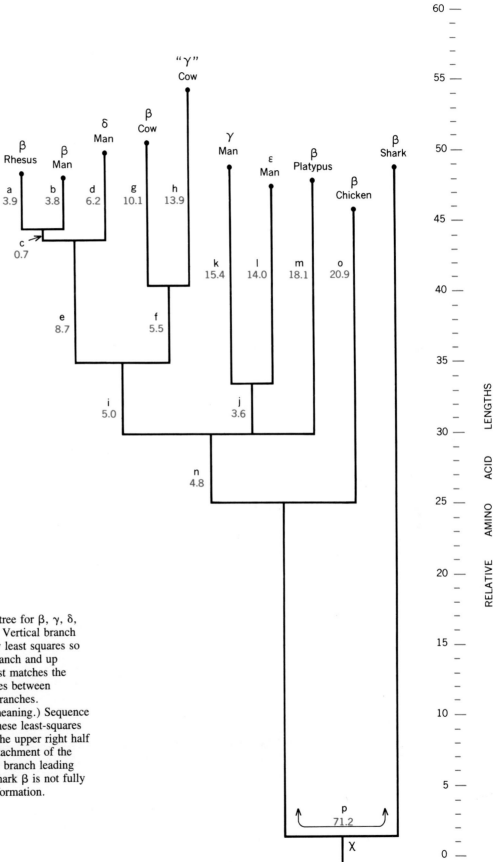

Figure 3.9 Ideally additive tree for β, γ, δ, and ε hemoglobin sequences. Vertical branch lengths have been adjusted by least squares so that the distance down one branch and up another (colored numbers) best matches the observed number of differences between sequences connected by the branches. (Horizontal distance has no meaning.) Sequence differences calculated using these least-squares branch lengths are shown in the upper right half of Table 3.4. The point of attachment of the continuation branch, *x*, to the branch leading from all other sequences to shark β is not fully defined without additional information.

solution to 45 equations in 16 unknowns. However, a convenient hand-calculator approach is to solve isolated subtrees first, and gradually expand the solution to the entire tree. In Figure 3.9 it is not difficult to obtain a best average set of values for variables $a, b, c,$ and d in one cluster, g and h in another, and $e + f$ connecting them. With these seven values held fixed, best average solutions can be found for the other variables working down the branches of the tree. This approximate solution then can be improved by least-squares methods. This approach leads to the branch lengths shown by colored numbers in Figure 3.9. As a check, the differences between sequences that would result from these branch lengths can be calculated and compared with the original observed differences. This has been done in the upper right half of Table 3.4, above the matrix diagonal. The observed and calculated differences have a root-mean-square (rms) discrepancy of only 2.5. As another measure of agreement, if observed and calculated differences are plotted against one another and a straight line is fitted to the points by linear regression, the slope is 1.0003 and the linear regression coefficient is 0.995. In the two largest individual discrepancies, the β chicken versus β cow comparison suggests that distance $n + o$ should be 8.7 units longer, but the β chicken versus human ε comparison suggests that it should be 6.3 units shorter; the other six β chicken comparisons favor the branch lengths shown. All other individual discrepancies throughout the table are 4 units or less.

With these error limits in mind, can any of the inequalities in branch lengths in Figure 3.9 be given sensible and statistically likely evolutionary interpretations? It would appear that more of the changes between β and "γ" (fetal) chains of cow since they diverged have taken place in the fetal gene. Although the difference in branch length, 3.8, is close to the rms error of 2.5, the hypothesis is plausible. The ancestral molecule would have been an adult type with DPG sensitivity, and the change in protein function would have occurred in the fetal line. The β chain presumably was already well adapted for interactions with the α chain and for its physiological role. Most of the adjustments leading to a fetal hemoglobin with increased oxygen affinity in the presence of DPG would have to occur in the gene for the new chain, and this is just what Figure 3.9 shows. In contrast, the difference in branch lengths of human β and γ up from their common connection point is only 0.8, entirely within experimental errors.

The tree just constructed fits the data well, but it has two fundamental flaws, both of which can be corrected to a degree:

1. Sequence differences have been measured in amino acid changes, implying that each exchange of one amino acid for another has the same evolutionary weight. Mutations, however, occur at the level of the DNA codons, and we know from the genetic code that some amino acid exchanges cannot be achieved without altering two of the bases, or even all three. We should properly be working with DNA sequences, not amino acid sequences, but until recently such DNA sequences have not been generally available.

2. The observed difference between two species seriously underestimates the actual number of genetic events that have occurred in the branches leading to present-day species from a common ancestral branch point. Repeated changes at the same amino acid position will not be seen just by comparing modern sequences. Even worse problems arise from the degeneracy of the genetic code (Figure 3.10). "Silent" mutations that lead from one codon to another for the same amino acid (UUG–leucine to CUG–leucine, for example) will be invisible, even though they are as legitimate evolutionary events as the replacement of tryptophan (UGG) by arginine (CGG).

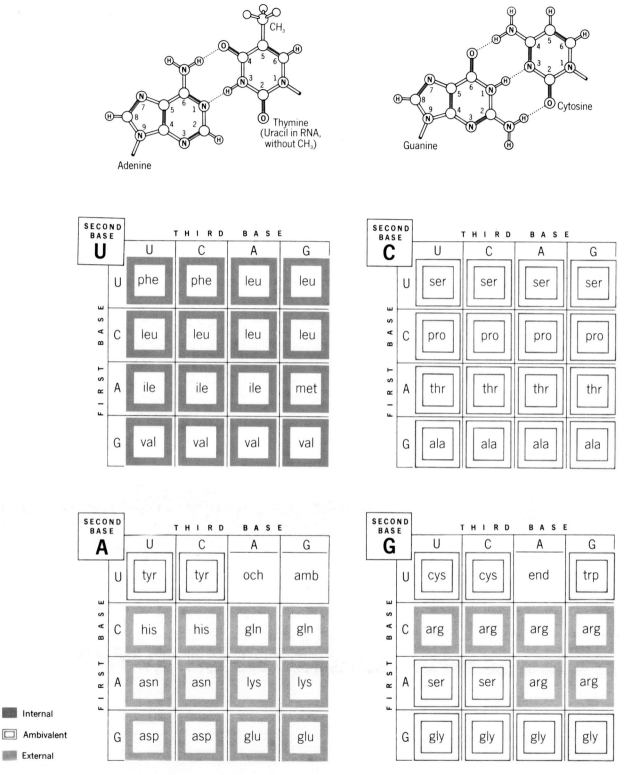

Figure 3.10 The genetic code. Each amino acid in a protein chain is coded by three consecutive bases in the DNA or the messenger RNA that is derived from it. With four possible bases at each position, A—C—G—T (or A—C—G—U in RNA), there are $4^3 = 64$ possible coding triplets or codons. Three are used as "stop" signals during protein synthesis at the ribosomes: UAA, UAG, and UGA. The other 61 are used to specify the 20 amino acids. This makes the code redundant, with more than one codon for several of the amino acids. For example, tryptophan is specified only by UGG, but arginine can be specified by six different triplet codons. The three functional categories of internal (color), ambivalent (uncolored), and external (gray) amino acids are as in Figure 1.8. Notice that the second base of a codon is the most influential in determining the functional type of amino acid, and that the third base often is irrelevant, the same amino acid being used no matter which of the four bases is present.

The first problem will vanish in a few years, when we have enough DNA sequences to use them instead of the amino acid sequences now available. In the past ten years, starting essentially from zero, more than 500,000 nucleotides have been sequenced. In the meantime, a partial solution is obtained by counting the *minimum* number of base changes needed to go from one amino acid to another using the most favorable choice of codons. Instead of working with total amino acid changes between two sequences, one can use minimal DNA base changes (31, 32). Figure 3.11 shows one pictorial form of the conversion matrix between amino acid changes and minimal base changes (33). Amino acid interconversions that require a change in all three bases are scored in the matrix by a gray square, those that demand at least two base changes are marked by a colored square, and those that can be accomplished with only a single change are indicated by specifying which base is altered: 1, 2, or 3. With the sequences and this matrix in hand, it is a straightforward computer conversion to replace amino acid differences by minimal base changes, and this has been done in most evolutionary studies to date.

This conversion matrix also is a good way of illustrating the important principle of the built-in conservatism of the genetic code: It is structured so that one or two base changes tend to lead to amino acids of similar properties, whereas radical alterations in amino acid character require two or three base changes. The genetic code is a "fail-safe" system, designed to damp down the effects of base mutations on the resulting polypeptide chains. The external, ambivalent, and internal categories of amino acids in Figures 3.10 and 3.11 are derived from their occurrence in known protein structures, and reflect mainly the

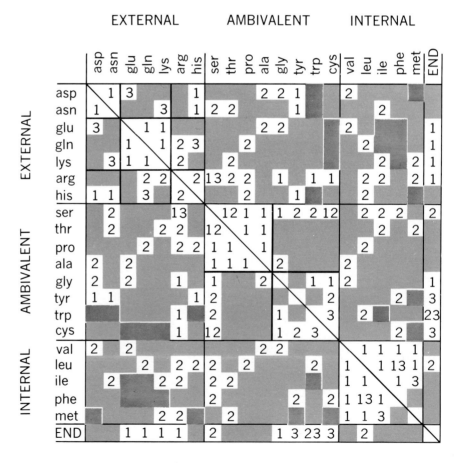

Figure 3.11 Minimal base change matrix for amino acid changes. Amino acid replacements requiring a change in all three bases of the codon are identified by grey squares, and those requiring at least two base changes are marked with colored squares. Numbers 1, 2, and 3 indicate single-base interconversions that can be accomplished by changing the first, second, or third base of the codon. If this can be accomplished in two ways, both numbers are given. (From Reference 30.)

polarity or hydrophobicity of the side chains. Changes within one category require one or two base mutations, whereas changes betwcen categories, especially external and internal, generally require two and frequently three base mutations. Among the single-base changes, the scarcity of 3's in the matrix is a reflection of the near-degeneracy of the third codon position—the fact that the choice of amino acid frequently is independent of the identity of the third base. The figure 2 is more common than 1 in the off-diagonal blocks of the matrix that represent shifts between categories of amino acid. This reflects the importance of the middle base in determining the nature of the resulting amino acid (Figure 3.10): U and C for nonpolar, or A and G for polar residues. Within the external amino acids, Asp-Asn, Glu-Gln-Lys, and Arg-His make up close-knit subsets, as do Ser-Thr-Pro-Ala in the ambivalent residues, and all five internal residues. Whether these have any significance in the history of the evolution of the genetic code itself is a question worth considering.

The second problem mentioned earlier, the lack of information about repeated changes at the same amino acid position, is a little more difficult to handle. The simplest procedure is to assume a random, Poisson distribution of mutations, and to correct the observed number of changes on this basis. This procedure has been followed in quite a few studies (18, 32, 34–36). The derivation of the correction factor to convert changes seen to changes that occurred is straightforward. Suppose that the rate at which mutational changes in a sequence has occurred is m changes per 100 positions in a given time period—that is, the intrinsic mutation frequency is $m/100 = M$ per residue. If the probability that a specific position will come through unscathed during this time period is $P_0 = k$ (a constant, to be evaluated), then the probability that it will instead be hit by one change is $P_1 = kM$. The probability of two successive changes occurring (of which only one would be seen) is $P_2 = kM^2/2$. The division by 2 is necessary because it makes no difference which of the two mutations came first; we are only interested in the likelihood that a total of two mutations would occur at the given position during the time period. The probability of three successive changes is $P_3 = kM^3/3!$, where again the denominator, $3! = 3 \cdot 2 \cdot 1 = 6$, is the number of ways of randomly permuting the order of three unlabeled entities (the three mutations). In general, the probability that x mutations have occurred at the same position is $P_x = kM^x/x!$. The constant, k, can be evaluated if we recognize that the probability that *something* happened, either no mutation or 1, 2, 3, . . . mutations, is equal to 1:

$$1 = P_0 + P_1 + P_2 + P_3 + \cdots = k\left(1 + M + \frac{M^2}{2!} + \frac{M^3}{3!} + \cdots\right) = ke^{+M}$$

Hence $k = e^{-M}$, and the general expression for the probability of x random mutational events taking place at one locus, given an intrinsic frequency M, is

$$P_x = e^{-M}\frac{M^x}{x!}$$

This is termed a Poisson distribution.

What is the probability that *at least one* mutation has occurred at the chosen site during the given time period, if it is a matter of indifference whether the true number of changes was really 1, 2, 3, 4, or more? This probability, N, is the sum of all probabilities, 1, less the probability that zero mutations occurred:

$$N = 1 - P_0 = 1 - e^{-M}$$

If 100 amino acids are chosen as a convenient data set for comparisons, then the occurrence of $m = 100\ M$ mutations randomly distributed along the sequence would lead to $n = 100\ N$ sequence changes that could be seen at the end of the given time period, where:

$$n/100 = 1 - e^{-m/100}$$

Hence an observed n change per 100 residues should be corrected to m mutational events, where:

$$m = -100 \ln\left(1 - \frac{n}{100}\right)$$

This relationship between mutations occurring, m, and number of changes seen, n, is plotted in Figure 3.12. The difference is small for 1 to 15 changes, but becomes appreciable above that point.

A simple Poisson correction to amino acid differences is not good enough because it overlooks both the degeneracy of the genetic code for a given change, and the existence of silent base mutations that do not change the amino acid sequence. A Poisson correction to the actual DNA sequence differences would be satisfactory, if we knew these differences, but applying the correction to the minimal mutation differences again underestimates the number of evolutionary events. Holmquist has developed a more elaborate statistical method to circumvent this (37–40). This method has the effect roughly of lowering the Poisson curve of Figure 3.12 at higher m values, thus increasing m for a given n, or increasing the number of presumed mutational events that lie behind an observed sequence difference. Dayhoff has achieved much the same thing by an empirical computer study, generating probability matrices for amino acid changes after successive mutational steps, using pairwise amino acid replacement frequency tables derived from an analysis of large numbers of real sequences (12). The empirical correction curve is compared with the Poisson correction in Figure 3.12. The Dayhoff PAM is a scrambled acronym for Accepted Point Mutation, and has the same meaning as the quantity m if 100 amino acids are being compared.

Even the Dayhoff empirical correction has been criticized as inadequately accounting for repeated or silent mutations, and for the fact that one can work only with inferred minimal base differences rather than true differences. Two

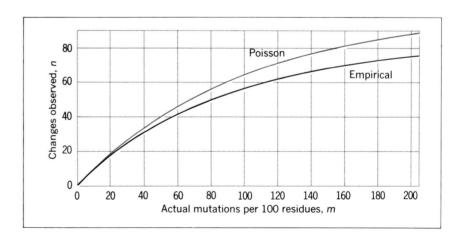

Figure 3.12 Correction curves for multiple mutations at the same position. If n sequence differences are observed, then m mutational events must be assumed to have occurred. Poisson = simple Poisson statistical correction. Empirical = correction derived by Dayhoff from empirical computer modeling studies (12).

entirely different and more elaborate approaches have been used to correct for this, and it is encouraging that they appear to converge on a common answer. Holmquist's *statistical or stochastic method,* mentioned earlier, is an elaboration of Poisson statistics that takes into explicit account multiple mutations at the same base site and within the same codon, the degeneracy of the code itself, and the possibility of back mutations. It places an approximate upper bound on the total number of mutational events that have occurred. In contrast, the *maximum parsimony method* attempts an actual reconstruction of ancestral sequences that require the fewest overall mutations to explain the observed present-day sequences. It was developed by Fitch (41–47), and has been elaborated and extended by Goodman and Moore (48–52). In its simplest form it merely

Figure 3.13 Augmented parsimony phylogenetic tree of the globin family. Numerals in roman type give the number of mutational events in each leg of the tree necessary to explain the present-day sequences in the most parsimonious manner. Italic numerals above them are values after augmentation to take into account invisible events: superimposed mutations at the same locus, silent mutations involving degeneracy of the genetic code, and back mutations to the original amino acid. Open and closed diamonds at branch points indicate certain and postulated gene duplications, respectively. The vertical axis is the age in millions of years for various branch points as deduced from the paleontological record and is not derived from the sequences themselves. This is in contrast to trees such as Figures 3.5 and 3.9, where the vertical axis measures *only* the degree of sequence difference, not elapsed time. For simplicity, all the mammalian species have been represented only by a single branch in myoglobin and in α and β hemoglobin. See also Figure 3.14. (From Reference 50.)

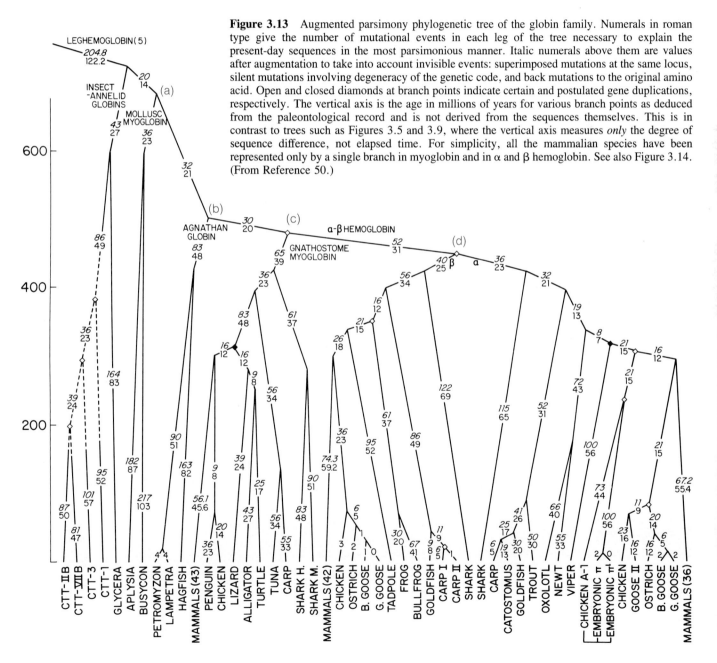

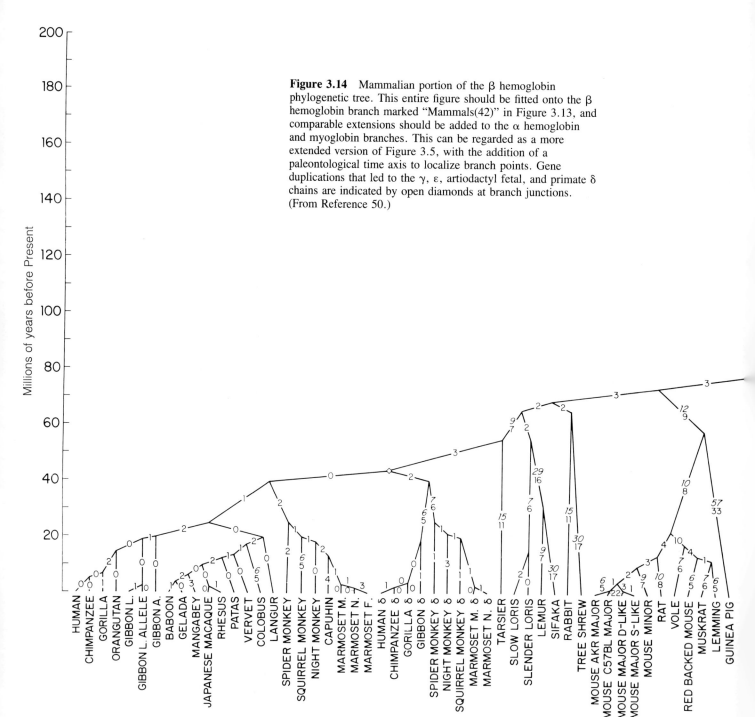

Figure 3.14 Mammalian portion of the β hemoglobin phylogenetic tree. This entire figure should be fitted onto the β hemoglobin branch marked "Mammals(42)" in Figure 3.13, and comparable extensions should be added to the α hemoglobin and myoglobin branches. This can be regarded as a more extended version of Figure 3.5, with the addition of a paleontological time axis to localize branch points. Gene duplications that led to the γ, ε, artiodactyl fetal, and primate δ chains are indicated by open diamonds at branch junctions. (From Reference 50.)

produces the optimum set of ancestral base sequences for a given phylogenetic tree, but the method also has been extended to finding the optimal tree or trees themselves. After establishing the maximum parsimony history of a set of sequences, Goodman and Moore then attempt to correct for missing mutational events by augmenting the branch lengths of their phylogenetic tree so that sparsely populated branches (with few sequences) have as high an average density of mutations as the most populated branches. It is these augmented distances (AD) that have been found to approach the random evolutionary hits (REH) of the stochastic theory in studies of globins (54) and cytochrome *c* (55).

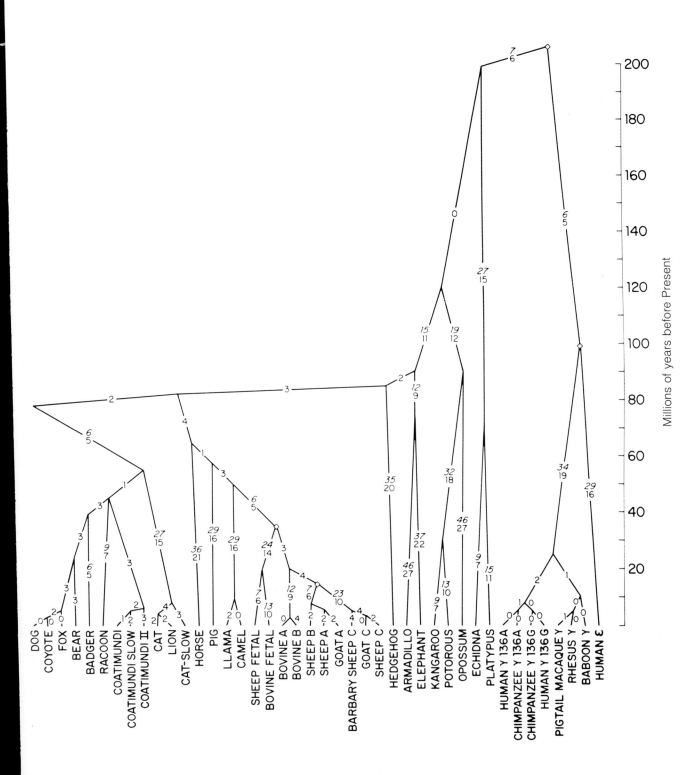

A phylogenetic tree of the globins based on the augmented parsimony approach is shown in Figures 3.13 and 3.14. It is a quantitative version of the schematic tree in Figure 3.6, with the addition of more species. It differs from the trees in Figures 3.5 and 3.9 in one important respect: The vertical axis no longer measures the degree of sequence difference. Rather, it is a *time* axis based on divergence dates as established by classical paleontological methods. The tree in Figure 3.13 shows very clearly the separation of the myoglobin, α, and β hemoglobin families, and their independent history of species divergence thereafter. In only one respect can it be seriously faulted: the branching off of Agnatha (lamprey) globin prior to the myoglobin/hemoglobin split. If the lower left half of the difference matrix in Table 3.3 is examined, sea lamprey globin appears to be slightly more different from α and β hemoglobin (mean and standard deviation of 120.8 ± 3.7 changes) than the various myoglobins are from these same hemoglobins (117.2 ± 4.9 changes). But these raw differences are deceptive: Table 3.1 shows that lamprey globin has an eight amino acid chain beginning that is absent from all other globins, except for a very different initial sequence in shark α hemoglobin. The all-differences counting method in this half of the table counts these as eight separate changes, even though they all probably resulted from a single crossover event or change in initiator codon. Similarly, it probably is excessive to count the lamprey deletion at the GH corner as nine separate evolutionary events. When the chains being compared have widespread insertions and deletions, then the all-differences count becomes inaccurate.

The upper right half of Table 3.3 gives only the common differences, or the number of amino acid changes at those positions along the chain that are possessed by both species being compared. A deletion in either chain causes that position to be rejected from the count. Hence these numbers measure the degree of similarity or difference in portions of chain that the two molecules have in common. With this method of counting, lamprey globin is seen to be virtually as close to the other α and β hemoglobins as the shark hemoglobin chains are (92.7 ± 6.0 and 88.7 ± 5.0 changes, respectively). In contrast, lamprey globin is much less related to the various myoglobin chains (101.7 ± 1.4 changes). The lamprey chain definitely is a good hemoglobin, even though not yet differentiated into α and β chains. As confirmation of this interpretation, a myoglobin has been isolated from lamprey heart, although it has not been sequenced at the time of writing (56). However, with this one exception, an interchange of branch points *b* and *c*, Figures 3.13 and 3.14 become an excellent illustration of the evolution of the globin family. Other trees for individual hemoglobin and myoglobin chains can be found in references 53 and 57–59.

3.6   THE CLOCK HYPOTHESIS

One of the most hotly debated questions in molecular evolution over the past decade has been that of the "molecular clock"—whether the *average* rate of accumulation of sequence changes over geological time has been effectively constant for a given protein. The rate of change in sequence is a function of two factors: the intrinsic rate at which mutations occur in the DNA of the gene, and the likelihood that a change will be accepted because it is either beneficial or at least harmless, rather than being weeded out as deleterious. There may be real differences in mutation rates between different genes, but so little is known about this that most attention has been focused on the second part: the acceptability of the mutations in a properly functioning protein. No one would deny that short-term fluctuations in rates of acceptance of mutations can occur, and the apparently faster rate of change in the bovine fetal gene after it diverged from bovine β may be a borderline example. Different local rates of change have been reported in various branches of both the hemoglobin and myoglobin trees (50, 53, 57). Whenever a gene has duplicated in such a way that one daughter gene is producing the original protein while the other is making a variant that is being put to a slightly different use, one might expect to find faster sequence changes in the second gene because of altered selection pressures. But on a longer time scale, is there any practical meaning to the concept of an *average* rate of change of sequence for a given protein, and does this tell us anything about the mechanism of sequence change?

Figure 3.15 shows the average number of amino acid differences between species on different sides of an evolutionary branch point, after simple Poisson correction, plotted against the time in the past at which that branch occurred as revealed by the fossil record. Of course many more sequences were used than those in Table 3.1. Of the 186 vertebrate globin sequences available, a set of 93 was selected in order to give a reasonably uniform distribution among phyla

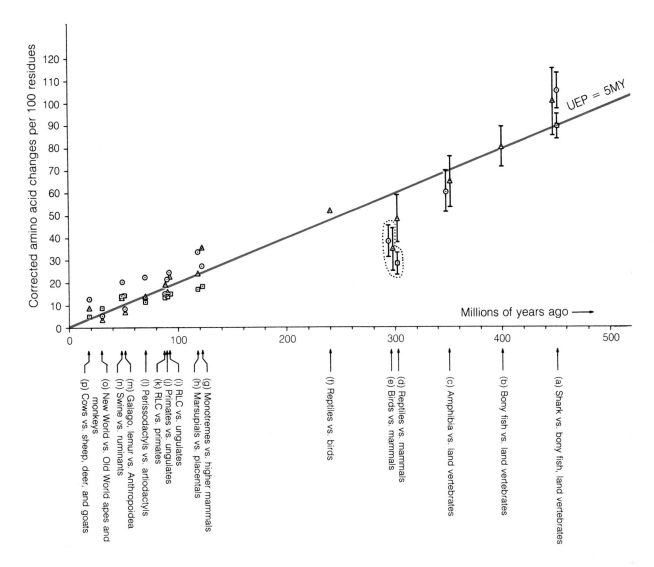

Figure 3.15 Rates of change of hemoglobin and myoglobin chains. The Poisson-corrected average number of amino acid differences between species on two sides of each evolutionary branch point is plotted against the time in the past at which that branch occurred as deduced from the paleontological record. (Data from Table 3.5.) Vertical error bars for the older divergence points extend over ±2 standard deviations, or to the 95% confidence level. Triangles represent α hemoglobin, circles are β hemo-globin, and squares are myoglobin. The straight line is the best linear regression fit to all data points. The slope of the line defines an average Unit Evolutionary Period (UEP), the time for a 1% sequence difference to accumulate between branches. For all three globin chains, UEP = 5 million years. (RLC = rodents, lago-morphs (rabbits), and carnivores. Adapted and extended from Reference 18.)

without excessive emphasis on mammals (Appendix 3.2). The mean differences used to prepare Figure 3.15 are given in Table 3.5, along with their reduction to a base of 100 amino acids, Poisson correction, and the assumed paleontological dates. The latter are not the times in the past at which representative species on both sides of a given branch point are abundantly represented in the fossil record, but are the older times at which the ancestors of the two groups of species probably diverged from a common stock (18, 60). The straight line drawn through these points is the result of a linear regression analysis, and seems a reasonable fit to the data. The slope of this line defines what Margoliash and Smith (35) have termed the Unit Evolutionary Period (UEP): the length of time for sequences on two sides of a common branch point to develop a 1% sequence difference. This figure is roughly 5 million years for each of the three globin chains.

Kimura has defined a rate constant for amino acid replacement along a single line of development: k_{aa} is the fractional rate of change per amino acid (aa) site per year (36). The two measures of change are reciprocally related:

$$k_{aa} \text{ (changes per year per site)} = \frac{1}{200 \text{ UEP (years)}}$$

The UEP of 5×10^6 years for the globins corresponds to a value of $k_{aa} = 10^{-9}$ amino acid changes per site per year. A similar treatment for the protein with the next most extensive sequence data set, the respiratory electron-transfer protein cytochrome *c*, yields a UEP of just over 20 million years (18), or a value of $k_{aa} = 0.25 \times 10^{-9}$ amino acid changes per site per year. Other proteins, for which fewer sequences are available for comparison, yield UEP values ranging from 0.7 million years (snake toxins and fibrinopeptides) to 500 million years (histones) (12, 18, 61). In general, the most slowly changing proteins are those that interact with other large macromolecules, such as histones and to a lesser degree cytochrome *c*, and members of organized multienzyme systems such as the glycolytic pathway. The more rapidly changing sequences are those for proteins or polypeptides that interact with smaller molecules or have less well defined functions. It seems to be a general principle that proteins with more finely drawn specifications, whether because they have an intricate structure or because they interact in a complex manner with other molecules, will be less tolerant of random mutational sequence changes. They accumulate acceptable changes more slowly, and hence will have a longer UEP.

One striking anomaly in Figure 3.15 should be mentioned, since it is present in all three globin chains, and to a lesser extent in cytochrome *c* as well. The bird versus mammal split (error bars surrounded by dotted lines in Figure 3.15) seems much too ancient—that is, bird and mammal sequences seem to be closer to one another than they have a right to be, assuming the same divergence time as for reptiles. Birds and mammals are both warm-blooded orders that evolved independently from reptiles. It usually has been assumed that the mammalian line split off from other reptiles early, and that the bird versus reptile split occurred later in the reptilian line, as drawn in Figure 3.16a. If so, then bird and reptile sequences should be equally distant from those of mammals. Instead, the average bird versus mammal differences are only 72% of the reptile (snake) versus mammal differences in α hemoglobin, and 65% in cytochrome *c*. (No data for reptilian β hemoglobin or myoglobin are available at the time of writing.) If the bird versus mammal divergence time is set at 300 million years ago as for reptiles versus mammals, then the bird versus mammal points fall well below the best

TABLE 3.5 RAW AND CORRECTED AMINO ACID SEQUENCE DIFFERENCES, AND SPECIES DIVERGENCE TIMES FOR FIGURE 3.15

Comparison[a]	Chain[b]	Number[c]	Raw differences[d]	Differences per 100 amino acids[d]	Poisson corrected differences[d,e]	Divergence date (MY)[f]
a. Shark vs. bony vertebrates	α	31	89.2 ± 4.0	63.3 ± 2.8	100.2 ± 7.6	450
	β	33	95.1 ± 2.0	65.1 ± 1.4	105.2 ± 4.0	"
	M	26	90.3 ± 1.7	59.0 ± 1.1	89.2 ± 2.7	"
b. Bony fish vs. land vertebrates	α	58	70.9 ± 3.1	50.3 ± 2.2	69.9 ± 4.4	400
c. Amphibia vs. land vertebrates	α	28	67.1 ± 4.2	47.6 ± 3.0	64.6 ± 5.7	350
	β	32	66.0 ± 3.7	45.2 ± 2.5	60.1 ± 4.6	"
d. Reptiles vs. mammals	α	25	53.9 ± 4.6	38.2 ± 3.3	48.1 ± 5.3	300
e. Birds vs. mammals	α	25	41.2 ± 4.8	29.2 ± 3.4	34.5 ± 4.8	300
	β	31	46.0 ± 3.5	31.5 ± 2.4	37.8 ± 3.5	"
	M	25	37.5 ± 2.7	24.5 ± 1.8	28.1 ± 2.4	"
f. Reptiles vs. birds	α	1	57	40.4	51.8	240
g. Monotremes vs. higher mammals	α	66	42.2 ± 3.6	29.9 ± 2.6	35.5 ± 3.7	120
	β	58	35.2 ± 3.7	24.1 ± 2.5	27.6 ± 3.3	"
	M	24	25.5 ± 3.7	16.7 ± 2.4	18.3 ± 2.9	"
h. Marsupials vs. placentals	α	21	30.0 ± 3.7	21.3 ± 2.6	24.0 ± 3.3	120
	β	54	41.9 ± 4.1	28.7 ± 2.8	33.8 ± 3.9	"
	M	44	24.0 ± 4.8	15.7 ± 3.1	17.1 ± 3.7	"
i. Rodents, lagomorphs, and carnivores vs. ungulates	α	28	28.2 ± 4.1	20.0 ± 2.9	22.3 ± 3.5	90
	β	27	31.6 ± 5.5	21.6 ± 3.8	24.3 ± 4.8	"
	M	20	21.4 ± 5.8	14.0 ± 3.8	15.1 ± 4.4	"
j. Primates vs. ungulates	α	70	20.3 ± 2.5	14.4 ± 1.8	15.5 ± 2.1	90
	β	117	28.1 ± 4.1	19.2 ± 2.8	12.3 ± 3.5	"
	M	12	19.9 ± 7.1	13.0 ± 4.6	13.9 ± 5.3	"
k. Rodents, lagomorphs, and carnivores vs. primates	α	40	24.7 ± 4.8	17.5 ± 3.4	19.3 ± 4.1	90
	β	39	20.2 ± 5.9	13.8 ± 4.0	14.9 ± 4.6	"
	M	15	19.4 ± 3.1	12.7 ± 2.0	13.6 ± 2.3	"
l. Perissodactyls vs. artiodactyls	α	6	18.0 ± 0.9	12.8 ± 0.6	13.7 ± 0.7	70
	β	14	29.4 ± 4.4	20.1 ± 3.0	22.4 ± 3.8	"
	M	3	16.3 ± 1.5	10.7 ± 1.0	11.3 ± 1.1	"
m. Galago, lemur vs. Anthropoidea	α	7	9.1 ± 1.6	6.5 ± 1.1	6.7 ± 1.2	51
	β	8	11.9 ± 1.1	8.2 ± 0.7	8.6 ± 0.8	"
	M	9	20.4 ± 2.2	13.3 ± 1.4	14.3 ± 1.6	"
n. Swine vs. ruminants	α	5	17.8 ± 1.9	12.6 ± 1.3	13.4 ± 1.5	50
	β	6	26.7 ± 4.6	18.3 ± 3.2	20.2 ± 3.9	"
	M	2	20.0 ± 4.2	13.1 ± 2.7	14.0 ± 3.1	"
o. New World vs. Old World apes and monkeys	α	10	4.7 ± 0.9	3.3 ± 0.6	3.4 ± 0.6	30
	β	12	6.8 ± 1.7	4.7 ± 1.2	4.8 ± 1.3	"
	M	2	12.5 ± 2.1	8.2 ± 1.4	8.6 ± 1.5	"
p. Cows vs. sheep, deer, and goats	α	4	11.2 ± 1.0	7.9 ± 0.7	8.2 ± 0.8	18
	β	4	18.2 ± 6.6	12.5 ± 4.5	13.4 ± 5.1	"
	M	1	8	5.2	5.3	"

[a]Sequences compared are listed in Appendix 3.2 of this chapter. *All differences* have been used as defined in Table 3.3, rather than *common differences*, but the distinction is minor within any one globin chain type.

[b]α = α hemoglobin; β = β hemoglobin; M = myoglobin.

[c]The total number of individual comparisons of species on two sides of a branch point. If 9 ungulate sequences are individually compared with 13 primate sequences, then the number would be 117.

[d]Average differences from all pairwise comparisons on two sides of a branch are given in the form of: Mean ± standard deviation.

[e]Poisson correction:

$$\frac{m}{100} = -\ln\left(1 - \frac{n}{100}\right),$$

where m changes per 100 amino acids are inferred to have occurred when n changes are actually observed. Correction to standard deviation:

$$\sigma_m = \sigma_n \exp\left(\frac{m}{100}\right)$$

[f]Paleontological dates for the various divergence points are taken from references 18 and 60. MY = million years ago.

Figure 3.16 Alternative phylogenetic trees for birds and mammals. (a) The conventional tree, which makes birds and reptiles equidistant from mammals. (b) A possible revision in which birds and mammals, although evolving independently from reptilian ancestors, are equally distant from modern snakes for which protein sequences are available. Although this revised tree would eliminate the bird–mammal paradox of Figure 3.15, it apparently is invalidated by the recent observation that the same paradox is observed when alligator myoglobin is compared with that of birds and mammals.* Alligators and crocodiles are certainly more closely related to birds than either is to mammals.

overall line. Alternatively, if the bird versus mammal points are shifted arbitrarily to the left until they fall on this line, then the calculated time of separation is only around 160 million years ago.*

This similarity of bird and mammal sequences may be an example of evolutionary *convergence* at the molecular level. Warm-blooded species, with their higher metabolic rates, may make similarly high demands on the molecules of their energy-production system, both those that help extract energy (cytochromes) and those that supply the oxygen (globins). Birds and mammals resemble one another not only in their regulation of body temperature, but in the development of comparable if different means of thermal insulation (feathers and fur), an active mode of life demanding acute senses and sufficient brainpower to process and use this sensory information, the ability to learn, and an extended period of care and instruction for their young. In many respects birds and mammals have evolved along parallel lines, and if we knew more about the relationships between macromolecular structure and metabolism, perhaps we could understand why some of their proteins should also have developed along similar lines.

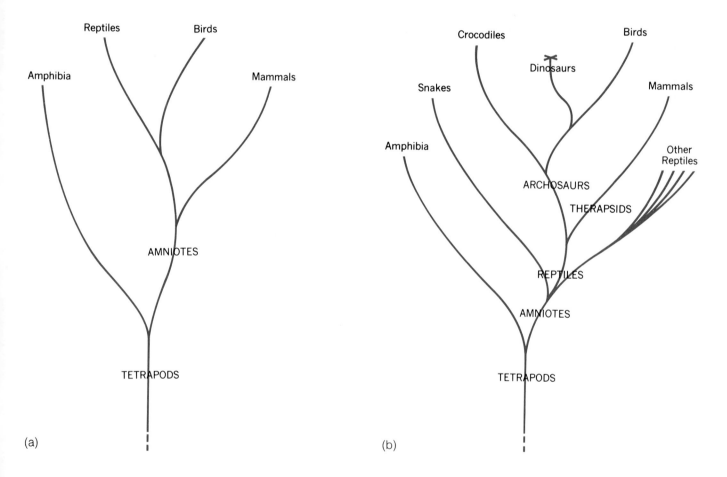

(a) (b)

---

*The more recent availability of an alligator myoglobin sequence intensifies the mammal–bird–reptile paradox. In a comparison of 27 mammals versus 2 birds (chicken and penguin), the mean difference and standard deviation between groups are 40.4 ± 3.8. Corresponding values for 27 mammals versus one reptile (alligator) are 55.6 ± 2.9, and those for two birds versus alligator are 51.0 ± 4.2. Once again, birds and mammals seem to be closer than they should be: the bird versus mammal differences are only 73% of the reptile versus mammal differences in myoglobins, uncannily close to the 72% for alpha hemoglobins.

TABLE 3.6 DIVERGENCE OF GLOBIN CHAIN TYPES

Comparison	Raw differences	Difference per 100 amino acids	Poisson corrected difference	Derived divergence date[a]	Geological era
1. 4 primate δ vs. 8 primate β	10.8 ± 2.2	7.4	7.7	36	Oligocene
2. Fetal cow vs. 4 cow, sheep β	14.3 ± 5.5	9.7	10.2	54	Eocene
3. Human γ vs. ε	30	20.5	22.9	116	Cretaceous
4. Human γ, ε vs. 29 mammalian β	39.2 ± 3.2	26.7	31.1	154	Jurassic
5. Human ζ vs. 27 α of snake or higher vertebrates	62.1 ± 3.1	42.3	55.0	274	Early Permian
6. 32 α family vs. 34 β family	88.9 ± 5.8	60.6	93.1	466	Ordovician
7. 27 myoglobins vs. 64 hemoglobins	115.4 ± 3.9	78.7	155	775	Precambrian

[a]In millions of years ago.

Another possible explanation must at least be considered. The idea has been advanced that birds evolved from the archosaurs (a group of small dinosaurs that learned to control their body temperature) and that feathers, like fur, evolved originally for thermal insulation rather than flight (62, 63). The argument as to how far back in the ancestral dinosaur line warm-bloodedness existed, although interesting, does not concern us here. But if the two reptilian lines that eventually developed temperature control, archosaurs for birds and therapsid reptiles for mammals, diverged from the ancestors of snakes before they went their own separate ways, then a tree such as Figure 3.16b would be correct, and modern birds and mammals would be more closely related than either is to present-day snakes. The observed differences in globin and cytochrome sequences would be accounted for. The question can be resolved only after more bird and reptilian sequences are available, but this may be one example of the way in which molecular information can help to clear up gaps in the paleontological record.

Figure 3.15, having been established using known paleontological dates for species divergences, now can be used to assign approximate dates to the gene duplications that are numbered 1–7 in Figure 3.6. This assignment is entirely independent of the particular type of empirical, Poisson, REH, or parsimony correction that might have been applied to the observed differences, as long as the same correction is applied to both sequence differences and gene divergence differences. Table 3.6 shows how the dates of gene divergence can be established using Poisson-corrected differences and Figure 3.15. The answers are paleontologically reasonable: The β/δ split occurred around 36 million years ago during primate diversification, the bovine fetal gene developed from the β during the radiation of the artiodactyls in the Eocene, the embryonic ε gene split off from the fetal γ during the development of placental mammals in the Cretaceous, the fetal γ gene itself had its origin around 150 million years ago in the therapsid reptiles that would give rise to mammals (60, 64), and the α/β split itself occurred more than 450 million years ago during the development of sharks and bony fish. The separation of the embryonic ζ gene from the adult α also appears to be quite old, but we know too little about this gene to say whether the date given in the table is reasonable or not.

It is tempting to extrapolate the line in Figure 3.15 all the way back to the separation of myoglobin and hemoglobin genes, in order to assign a date to divergence point 7 in Figure 3.6. The resulting figure of 775 million years, however, seems much too large. Lamprey and the other Agnatha diverged from cartilaginous fish (sharks) and bony fish around 500 million years ago in the early Ordovician period (60). One could attempt to save the situation by claiming that hemoglobin and myoglobin descended from *different* examples of the multiple copies of globin genes possessed by the ancestral invertebrates, and that these multiple copies separated from one another 775 million years ago. Fitch (65) has drawn the important distinction between *orthologous* and *paralogous* genes in comparing sequences: In two species, orthologous genes are those that lie in a direct line of descent from *the same gene* in the nearest ancestor shared by both species, whereas paralogous genes are derived from different (although related) genes in the common ancestor. The horse β and human β hemoglobin genes are orthologous, whereas horse α and human β genes (or human α and β genes, for that matter) are paralogous. It is only valid to compare orthologous genes when studying phylogenetic relationships. A person who attempted to learn about the differentiation of primates and perissodactyls by comparing primate α chains with equine β chains would end up with nonsense.

As has been mentioned earlier, lamprey and invertebrates seem to contain several globin genes, which we now would term paralogous, whose actual divergence points lie in the unknown past. When we know the amino acid sequences of all six lamprey hemoglobins and the recently discovered lamprey myoglobin, and have similar data for the paralogous sets of globin genes of other invertebrates, then logical patterns may begin to emerge. At the moment, the extraordinarily ancient date of 775 million years for hemoglobin/myoglobin obtained by a literal application of the clock hypothesis might be salvaged by claiming that the myoglobin and hemoglobin genes of higher organisms developed from paralogous invertebrate genes. If this is true, then once the sequence data become available, we should be able to map these paralogous genes through the various invertebrates, in the way that one can map the myoglobin and α and β hemoglobin genes through the vertebrates.

Another possibility seems intuitively reasonable. If sequences tend to evolve more rapidly early in the history of a given protein, when it is as yet imperfectly adapted for its biological role (18), then one should expect to observe a more rapid sequence change in the early hemoglobins and myoglobins, followed by a "settling down" of changes as each protein became optimally adjusted for its own particular function. Under such circumstances a linear clock assumption would give a spuriously ancient date for the divergence of hemoglobin and myoglobin genes, as the 775-million-year figure would seem to indicate. With this model, the linear curve in Figure 3.15 should begin to assume an upward curvature at the extreme right, and the cluster of three error bars for the divergence of shark from bony fish suggests that this may be so. If, indeed, one fits the best linear regression line through points *a–e* in Figure 3.15 as a rough approximation to an upward slope at the oldest branch points, then the hemoglobin versus myoglobin divergence date falls from 775 million years to just under 600 million years, a much more believable figure. The data seem to demand one of two possible conclusions:

1. If the average rate of accumulation of globin sequence changes observed in Figure 3.15 has remained constant all the way back to the divergence of the ancestors of present-day myoglobin and hemoglobin genes, then myoglobin and hemoglobin are the products of paralogous genes that diverged 775 million years ago, long before the host species themselves diverged.

2. If the gene diversification occurred at the same time as the species whose sequences have been examined, then the initial rate of accumulation of sequence changes in the young hemoglobin and myoglobin genes was higher than the reasonably steady average value reflected in Figure 3.15.

The choice that is made depends to a degree on one's preconceived model preferences. Convinced neutralists will come down strongly in favor of the first option (66), whereas selectionists will argue equally fervently for the second option (53). Reality, as usual, probably will be found to lie somewhere in between the two extreme positions.

3.7 SELECTION VERSUS NEUTRAL DRIFT

The clock hypothesis has received so much attention because it bears on a fundamental dispute about the relative importance of two factors in molecular evolution: positive selection for advantageous changes versus random fixation of neutral mutations—selectionism versus neutralism. When amino acid sequences first were compared from an evolutionary viewpoint, it was assumed that the differences observed between two species were preserved by natural selection because each form was best, in some way, for its own species (67). Constant regions of sequence were explained as being so because they were essential to the basic functioning of the protein wherever found, so that chance mutations in the DNA for these regions would be ruthlessly weeded out. But variable regions were regarded as being equally essential for the *species* in which they occurred. An accidental mutation in an unimportant portion of sequence (if such existed) would be so outnumbered by the standard version in all the interbreeding individuals of the species (the gene pool) that it inevitably would be lost. "Neutral mutations cannot be preserved by natural selection" (35). A distinction was drawn between "function-specific" (invariant) and "species-specific" (variable) regions of the molecule. Where no logical explanation could be found for a sequence change between species, it was proposed that this change might represent a tailoring of the protein to the other macromolecules with which it had to interact, as cytochrome *c* must interact with its reductase and oxidase.

A radically different explanation was proposed by Kimura in 1968 (36, 68, 69) and King and Jukes the following year (70). They suggested that most DNA mutations might be selectively neutral—that is, the resulting protein with a changed amino acid might be able to function just as well as the original protein. By the principles of population genetics, such a random sequence change has a statistical probability of eventually displacing the original form, and the quotation in the previous paragraph is in fact incorrect. If we watch a population initially containing N individuals with $2N$ copies of a gene for a sufficiently long time, eventually the random drift of gene frequencies with mating will lead to the result that all the copies of that gene are descendants of just one of the original set (71, 72). (This might be called the "Adam principle.") The chance of this happening to any one of the $2N$ genes is $1/2N$. On the other hand, if the probability of any one gene experiencing a mutation during a particular generation is ν, then the total number of such mutations in that generation is $2N\nu$. The probability that one of these mutations will eventually become fixed as the dominant version of the gene in the distant future is

$$2N\nu \cdot \frac{1}{2N} = \nu$$

Hence the surprising conclusion that the probability of random fixation of a particular mutation is proportional to the intrinsic probability of the mutation, and is independent of population size! Large populations have more mutations, but a smaller chance that any one of them eventually will become dominant; small populations have fewer mutations, but each has a better chance of taking over. The two effects balance out.

Even if one were to begin with a mixture of roughly equal numbers of alleles (variants) of a given gene, the random sampling process inherent in each mating and new generation would ensure that the population eventually became skewed in distribution toward one allele or another. The smaller the population the more rapidly this occurs, with the rate varying as $1/2N$. All of the foregoing, of course, assumes that the selective fitness of all the alleles is identical, or that all changes are strictly neutral. If one of the alleles possessed even a slight positive advantage compared with the others, then over the generations it would tend to dominate. However, if the selection coefficient was small and the population was also small, then even an advantageous allele might be lost to a population by chance.

It is perhaps unfortunate that the neutralist ideas were introduced with the clever but emotion-laden label of "non-Darwinian evolution" (70). Genetic drift is just the limit of positive selection as the selective advantage of the new mutation approaches zero. The extreme selectionist and neutralist hypotheses, however, account for observed differences in protein sequences in different ways. The former would say that human and rhesus monkey α hemoglobin chains differ at position A6 because threonine is better for man at that point whereas serine is better for rhesus. The neutralist explanation would be that threonine and serine have exactly the same fitness at that location in the A helix, that a chance mutation occurred in the ancestor of one species, and that random genetic drift through the population in which the change occurred eventually led to its being fixed as the dominant form rather than being lost (which could equally well have happened). Man and rhesus have different residues at position A6, not because it matters to the operation of their hemoglobins, but because it does *not* matter.

A constant average rate of change of sequence with time for a protein is easier to explain by the neutralist theory than by positive selection. If certain regions of the molecule are "untouchable" because they are essential to the proper working of the protein, but other regions are unimportant and susceptible to random, neutral changes, then the rate at which these changes accumulate will be related to the relative numbers of essential and nonessential residues, or to the degree of selection pressure exerted on the molecule by the requirement that it work properly. A constant rate of accumulation of change implies only that the selection pressures on the resulting protein have been effectively constant over the same time period. This could happen, for example, if a protein were well adjusted to its role in a relatively unchanging functional setting. But by the selectionist theory, if a sequence changes only in response to positive selection pressure, then a constant observed rate of change over geological time requires that selection pressures themselves be *altering* at a constant rate, not that they be effectively constant. This seems a much more artificial and ad hoc principle, and convinced selectionists have tended to reject the clock hypothesis.

Figure 3.15 and others like it for other proteins tell us that (a) the clock is rather erratic on a short time scale, and (b) it may be gradually accelerating or decelerating over a sufficiently long time period. However, the rate for a given protein is sufficiently constant, and clocks for different proteins are sufficiently dissimilar, that the concept of a characteristic UEP for a protein is a useful one if not pushed too far. The actual evolutionary history of a gene contains both selective and neutral events. In principle one can define a selection coefficient for each possible amino acid exchange at every position of a protein, with the coefficient being positive if the change is advantageous, negative if deleterious, and zero if neutral. A mutation that replaced leucine in the interior of a protein by aspartic acid would have a large negative selection coefficient (unless the buried aspartic acid made possible some catalytic or other activity of the protein, as in the enzyme trypsin). On the other hand, the replacement of leucine by isoleucine or valine might have a coefficient very close to zero. Most interchanges of one acidic group for another, or one basic group for another, on the surface of a protein probably have very nearly zero selection coefficients. The scatter of aspartic or glutamic acid at positions A4 and B4 in Table 3.1 suggests that one is just about as good as the other. In contrast, the replacement of histidine at position FG3 of myoglobin by leucine had a positive selection coefficient in the genes that led to the α and β hemoglobin chains, since it facilitated the formation of dimers at the $\alpha_1\beta_2$ subunit interface. The value of the selection coefficient for a mutation depends on (a) the protein involved, (b) the exact position in that protein, and (c) the precise nature of the amino acid change. But if one allows the values of selection coefficients to range from large and positive (advantageous changes) through zero (neutral mutations) to large and negative (very deleterious or lethal mutations), then both selectionism and neutralism can be regarded as extreme viewpoints of a more general theory.

As has been mentioned earlier, positive selection might be expected to predominate during the early evolutionary development of a given protein, and neutral drift might be expected to take over once the protein had stabilized in a well-defined and relatively unchanging role. In addition, sequences in certain phylogenetic branches might change more rapidly or slowly than the overall average because of special selection pressures on that particular group of organisms. Goodman has claimed to see just such variations in the globins, cytochrome c, and other proteins (50, 53). With a set of presumed ancestral nucleotide sequences deduced by the maximum parsimony method, and with a most parsimonious tree whose branch points have been fixed by paleontological dates (Figures 3.13 and 3.14), one can examine individual branches of the tree for indications of unusually fast or slow variation.

With the globins, Goodman and co-workers see both a general effect and several specific ones. The general effect is a more rapid rate of sequence change early in the history of the globins, during the development from monomeric globins, through lamprey dimers, to a functional $\alpha_2\beta_2$ tetramer; a slower rate of change from the development of amniotes (reptiles and birds) to the beginning of the radiation of mammalian species; and a more rapid rate of change among the mammals. Although arrived at by quite a different approach, this interpretation amounts to fitting the globin data of Figure 3.15 with a three-step curve as in Figure 3.17. Whether such a procedure is legitimate or not is currently the subject of a spirited debate. Figure 3.17 demonstrates, however, that the trends that Goodman has called attention to *are* present in the globin data, and are not artifacts resulting from the maximum parsimony approach. The data in Figure 3.17 have been given only a simple Poisson correction, and the plot would be similar in appearance even if uncorrected sequence differences had been used.

The triphasic curve as drawn in Figure 3.17, although open to question, has three pragmatic advantages: It eliminates the bird versus mammal anomaly discussed earlier; it no longer requires the assumption of paralogous globin genes for myoglobin and hemoglobin or of an absurdly ancient myoglobin versus hemoglobin divergence date; and it can be given a simple interpretation in terms of natural selection, illustrating the principle that sequences change most rapidly when they are subject to intense selection pressures. The period of metazoan evolution up to 300 million years ago was one in which a primitive oxygen-binding monomer globin specialized into a storage protein and a transport protein, the transport protein itself evolved into a tetramer exhibiting subunit cooperativity and allosteric control by several small molecules, and the organ-

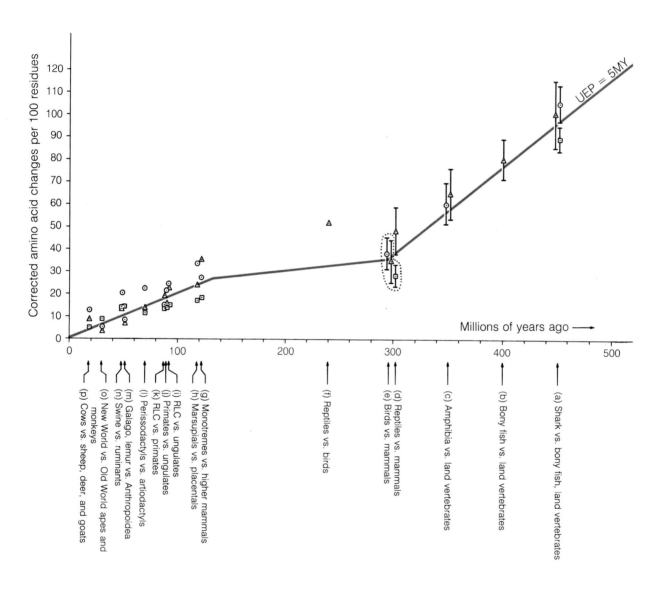

Figure 3.17 Alternative interpretation of globin rates of change. These are the identical data points of Figure 3.15 but reinterpreted in terms of three phases of globin evolution: rapid change during the evolution of a functional tetramer in air-breathing land vertebrates, slower change during the metabolically static era of reptiles, and rapid change once more during the radiation of warm-blooded mammals. The mammalian segment is identical with that of Figure 3.15, with a UEP of 5 million years. The reptilian segment has a UEP of 20 million years, and the earliest segment, obtained by linear regression fitting of points a–e, has a UEP of 2.5 million years. (See caption to Figure 3.15 for an explanation of symbols.)

isms that contained it evolved from simple aquatic metazoa into large, complex, land-based animals breathing atmospheric oxygen and distributing it among a great many specialized organs and tissues. Selection pressures must have been intense, both on the organisms and on many of their component proteins. In contrast, the achievement of a relatively stable ectothermic reptilian metabolism ushered in an era in which the demands for adaptation and change in the oxygen-circulating proteins would be relatively small, even though the reptiles were undergoing great anatomical diversification. Finally, beginning around 120 million years ago, new pressures on the oxygen-supplying and energy-extracting systems arose along with the development of endothermy and the radiation of mammals. As a consequence, the rate of change in the globin sequences increased once again as indicated in Figure 3.17. *Se non è vero, è ben trovato.*

Of the several specific local variations in globin sequence reported by Goodman, only two will be mentioned. Globin sequence changes within the primates appear to have slowed, coming nearly to a halt in the great apes and man. The amino acid sequences in man and chimpanzee are identical for α and β hemoglobins, cytochrome *c,* and fibrinopeptides A and B. Their myoglobins differ only by a single amino acid. Fossil evidence indicates that the ancestors of man and chimpanzee separated approximately 15 million years ago, so a globin UEP of 5 million years would lead one to expect

$$\frac{15}{5} \times \frac{150 \text{ aa}}{100 \text{ aa}} = 4.5$$

or around 4 to 5 amino acid differences per 150-residue globin chain. Why have all these proteins remained so constant in the line leading to *Homo sapiens?* This problem of primate evolution at the molecular level has been the subject of a special review volume (73), and a satisfactory answer remains to be found.

The other specific variation in globin sequence change pertains to the differential rate of change of different parts of the globin molecule during the evolution, first of a lamprey dimer, and then of a functional tetrameric hemoglobin. For the period from the invertebrate/vertebrate divergence to the last common ancestor of Agnatha and the bony fish (segment *a–b* in Figure 3.13), Goodman and co-workers deduce from their most parsimonious ancestral sequences that the region of the globin chain corresponding to the $\alpha_1\beta_2$ sliding-contact surface in the complete tetramer accumulated nucleotide sequence changes at four times the overall average rate for the molecule as a whole (50). During this same period, the positions corresponding to $\alpha_1\beta_1$ packing contacts only changed at the average whole-molecule rate. In contrast, during the period from the divergence of lamprey and bony fish to the α/β gene split (*b–d* in Figure 3.13), the $\alpha_1\beta_1$ packing-contact zones changed at nearly twice the average rate while the $\alpha_1\beta_2$ sliding-contact changes were virtually identical to the average. This is what one would expect if (a) the association of subunits in lamprey deoxyglobin is as proposed in Section 3.2—contacts between C helices and FG corners that are disrupted by oxygenation—and (b) the development of a two-state tetramer that held together even when oxygenated had to await the invention of the $\alpha_1\beta_1$ packing contacts that permitted a flexible joint between one pair of chains to hold together the switch region in the other. At each stage in the evolution of the tetramer, the portion of the molecule just being developed accepted base changes more rapidly than those regions that had already been developed or had yet to evolve. This argues for positive selection, rather than neutral fixation.

In sum, there seem to be moments in the evolution of a protein when its sequence changes are predominantly a consequence of natural selection, either to accelerate the development of a new or more efficient protein, or to hold fixed a particularly well-adjusted one under special circumstances. On the other hand, once a protein is well adapted for a particular role, it appears to settle down to a nearly constant rate of accumulation of sequence changes. It is hard to see this as anything other than the random fixation of near-neutral mutations (45, 69). The "clock" may be erratic, and it may run faster for a while after it is first wound up, but it seems to tick away fairly regularly if not jarred too often by changes in external conditions. The validity of the clock hypothesis has been affirmed by many investigators (12, 33, 36, 69) and denied by others (43–45, 49, 55), with occasional defections from one camp to the other (43, 47). The issue will not soon be resolved to everyone's satisfaction. But the question surely is not whether positive selection or neutral drift is *the* mode of production of sequence changes, but rather the *relative importance* of these two factors at different periods in protein evolution.

3.8 DARWIN'S MOLECULES

This chapter has concentrated on the evolution of the globins, since they are the subject of this book. Yet an equally comprehensive story can be presented today for the cytochromes *c,* and nearly as complete pictures can be drawn for other electron-transport proteins such as ferredoxins and flavodoxins, for the dehydrogenases and other enzymes of intermediary metabolism, immunoglobulins, chymotrypsin and most of the other digestive enzymes, hormones, nucleases, and even snake toxins. Furthermore, with the advance in DNA sequencing methods, that which has been achieved with amino acid sequences will soon be surpassed by the use of DNA sequences—not merely of genes for individual proteins, but of entire genomes hundreds of thousands of base pairs long.

It is always elegant to prove your theory using all the available evidence of the time; it is even more elegant to have your theory confirmed after the fact by new data that you never heard of. This is what has happened to Charles Darwin and Alfred Wallace and their theory of evolution. Darwin knew nothing of genetics; Gregor Mendel's important papers lay dormant and unappreciated in the Proceedings of the Natural History Society of Brno. Yet Mendelian genetics as developed in the first half of the twentieth century provided the mechanism for the variation and selection that Darwin proposed as being central to evolution. The fossil record that Darwin had to work with contained major gaps, including an almost complete blank in our own human lineage. But these gaps have been filled in to a remarkable degree since then, in a manner that has only confirmed our belief in the correctness of Darwin's vision. The explosion of new information on hominid fossils in East Africa since 1960 (74) has relegated the old phrase "the missing link" to the cabinet of Victorian curiosa along with "the chicken-and-egg paradox" and Sir Arthur Sullivan's "Lost Chord."

Perhaps the most remarkable new outpouring of evidence supporting evolution has come from the field of molecular biology, an area totally foreign to anything with which Darwin and Wallace were familiar. At the molecular level we now can describe in considerable detail the manner in which genetic information is stored, the several methods by which genetic variation arises, and how this variation is expressed in a way that makes it subject to natural selection. Equally striking is the observation (the subject of this chapter) that every organism carries around a miniature record of its evolutionary history in its proteins. Hemoglobin and myoglobin are as valid evidence in tracing phylogenetic relationships as are teeth and bones. But with the addition of molecular data to the study, the quantity of actual and potential new information bearing on evolutionary history has risen since 1960 by at least two orders of magnitude. The quantity of data available for study is limited today chiefly by the fatigue level of biochemists and the constraints of research funding.

Of course, even this mountain of new data will not *prove* the theory of evolution. One can never prove a theory in science; one can only demonstrate that it has not yet been disproven. But there comes a level of support at which the common sense of any unprejudiced observer leads to an acceptance of the theory as being beyond reasonable doubt. The theory of evolution in biology and the atomic theory in physics rest on equally secure data, and we understand considerably more about either of them than we do about the theory of gravitation. In the face of all of this evidence, one must reply to those few today who would emulate Bishop Samuel Wilberforce with neither his wit nor his learning: Either evolution is a fact, and is the way in which life diversified on our planet (and this can be regarded as either a nontheistic or a theistic process), or else the universe is inherently illogical and we are all the victims of a cosmic joke. Any other conclusion is logically untenable.

GENERAL REFERENCES

1. Sanger, F., and Tuppy, H., 1951. *Biochem. J.* 49:481–490.
2. Sanger, F., and Thompson, E. O. P., 1953. *Biochem. J.* 53:353–374.
3. Margoliash, E., Smith, E. L., Kreil, G., and Tuppy, H., 1961. *Nature* 192:1121–1127.
4. Braunitzer, G., Gehring-Muller, R., Hilschmann, N., Hilse, K., Hobom, G., Rudloff, V., and Wittmann-Liebold, B., 1961. *Z. Physiol. Chem.* 325:283–286.
5. Smyth, D. G., Stein, W. H., and Moore, S., 1963. *J. Biol. Chem.* 238:227–234.
6. Canfield, R., 1963. *J. Biol. Chem.* 238:2698–2707.
7. Keil, B., Prusik, Z., and Sorm, F., 1963. *Biochim. Biophys. Acta* 78:559–561.
8. Anfinsen, C. B., 1959. *The Molecular Basis of Evolution,* Wiley, New York.
9. Perutz, M. F., Rossmann, M. G., Cullis, A. F., Muirhead, H., Will, G., and North, A. T. C., 1960. *Nature* 185:416–422.
10. Kendrew, J. C., Dickerson, R. E., Strandberg, B. E., Hart, R. G., Davies, D. R., Phillips, D. C., and Shore, V. C., 1960. *Nature* 185:422–427.
11. Edmundson, A. B., 1965. *Nature* 205:883–887.
12. Dayhoff, M. O. *Atlas of Protein Sequence and Structure:* Vol. 5 (1972); Supplement 1 (1973); Supplement 2 (1976); Supplement 3 (1978). (All earlier volumes are superseded by Vol. 5 and its supplements.) *Nucleic Acid and Protein Sequence Databases.* Both Atlas and Databases are available from Georgetown University Medical Center, 3900 Reservoir Road N.W., Washington, D.C. 20007.
13. Thompson, E. O. P., 1980. In D. S. Sigman and M. A. B. Brazier (Eds.), *The Evolution of Protein Structure and Function,* Academic Press, New York, pp. 267–298.

14. Proudfoot, N. J., O'Connell, C., and Maniatis, T., 1980. Private communication.

15. Baralle, F. E., Shoulders, C. C., and Proudfoot, N. J., 1981. *Cell* 21:621–626.

16. Lehmann, H., and Huntsman, R. G., 1974. *Man's Haemoglobins* (2nd ed.), North-Holland Publishing Company, Amsterdam.

17. Hendrickson, W. A., 1973. *Biochim. Biophys. Acta* 310:32–38.

18. Dickerson, R. E., 1971. *J. Mol. Evolu.* 1:26–45.

19. Gale, R. E., Clegg, J. B., and Huehns, E. R., 1979. *Nature* 280:162–164.

20. Maniatis, T., Fritsch, E. F., Lauer, J., and Lawn, R. M., 1980. *Ann. Rev. Genetics* 14:145–178.

21. Efstratiadis, A., Posakony, J. W., Maniatis, T., Lawn, R. M., O'Connell, C., Spritz, R. A., DeRiel, J. K., Forget, B. G., Weissman, S. M., Slightom, J. L., Blechl, A. E., Smithies, O., Baralle, F. E., Shoulders, C. C., and Proudfoot, N. J., 1980. *Cell* 21:653–668.

22. Liebhaber, S. A., Goosens, M., and Kan, Y. W., 1980. *Proc. Natl. Acad. Sci. USA* 77:7054–7058.

23. Villeponteau, B., and Martinson, H., 1981. *Nucl. Acids Res.* 9:3731–3746.

24. Wood, W. G., 1976. *Brit. Med. Bull.* 32:282–287.

25. Jeffreys, A. J., Wilson, V., Wood, D., and Simons, J. P., 1980. *Cell* 21:555–564.

26. Jensen, E. Ø., Paludan, K., Hyldig-Nielsen, J. J., Jørgensen, P., and Marcker, K. A., 1981. *Nature* 291:677–679.

27. Jeffreys, A. J., 1979. *Cell* 18:1–10.

28. Gilbert, W., 1979. In *Eukaryotic Gene Regulation*, ICN–UCLA Symposium on Molecular and Cellular Biology, Vol. XIV. (R. Axel, T. Maniatis and C. F. Fox, Eds.), New York, Academic Press, p. 1012.

29. Slightom, J. L., Blechl, A. E., and Smithies, O., 1980. *Cell* 21:627–638.

30. Zimmer, E. A., Martin, S. L., Beverley, S. M., Kan, Y. W., and Wilson, A. C., 1980. *Proc. Natl. Acad. Sci. USA* 77:2158–2162.

31. Fitch, W. M., and Margoliash, E., 1967. *Science* 155:279–284.

32. Jukes, T. H., and Cantor, C. R., 1969. In H. N. Munro (Ed.), *Mammalian Protein Metabolism,* Vol. 3. Academic Press, New York, pp. 21–132.

33. Dickerson, R. E., 1971. *J. Mol. Biol.* 57:1–15.

34. Zuckerkandl, E., and Pauling, L., 1965. In V. Bryson and H. J. Vogel (Eds.), *Evolving Genes and Proteins,* Academic Press, New York, pp. 97–166.

35. Margoliash, E., and Smith, E. L., 1965. In V. Bryson and H. J. Vogel (Eds.), *Evolving Genes and Proteins,* Academic Press, New York, pp. 221–242.

36. Kimura, M., 1969. *Proc. Natl. Acad. Sci. USA* 63:1181–1188.

37. Holmquist, R., 1972. *J. Mol. Evolu.* 1:115–149.

38. Holmquist, R., Cantor, C., and Jukes, T., 1972. *J. Mol. Biol.* 64:145–161.

39. Holmquist, R., 1976. In M. Goodman, R. E. Tashian, and J. H. Tashian (Eds.), *Molecular Anthropology,* Plenum Press, New York, pp. 89–116.

40. Holmquist, R., Pearl, D., and Jukes, T. H., 1981. In M. Goodman (Ed.), *Macromolecular Sequences in Systematics and Evolutionary Biology,* Plenum Press, New York.

41. Fitch, W., 1971. *Syst. Zool.* 20:406–416.

42. Fitch, W. M., and Farris, J. S., 1974. *J. Mol. Evolu.* 3:263–278.

43. Langley, C. H., and Fitch, W. M., 1974. *J. Mol. Evolu.* 3:161–177.

44. Fitch, W. M., and Langley, C. H., 1976. *Fed. Proc.* 35:2092–2097.

45. Fitch, W. M., 1976. In F. J. Ayala (Ed.), *Molecular Evolution,* Sinauer Associates, Sunderland, Mass., pp. 160–178.
46. Fitch, W. M., and Langley, C. H., 1976. In M. Goodman, R. E. Tashian, and J. H. Tashian (Eds.), *Molecular Anthropology,* Plenum Press, New York, pp. 197–219.
47. Gillespie, J. H., and Langley, C. H., 1979. *J. Mol. Evolu.* 13:27–34.
48. Moore, G. W., Barnabas, J., and Goodman, M., 1973. *J. Theor. Biol.* 38:459–485.
49. Goodman, M., Moore, G. W., Barnabas, J., and Matsuda, G., 1974. *J. Mol. Evolu.* 3:1–48.
50. Goodman, M., Moore, G. W., and Matsuda, G., 1975. *Nature* 253:604–608.
51. Goodman, M., 1976. In F. J. Ayala (Ed.), *Molecular Evolution,* Sinauer Associates, Sunderland, Mass., pp. 141–159.
52. Moore, G. W., 1976. In M. Goodman, R. E. Tashian, and J. H. Tashian (Eds.), *Molecular Anthropology,* Plenum Press, New York, pp. 117–137.
53. Goodman, M., 1981. *Progr. Biophys. Mol. Biol.* 38:105–164.
54. Holmquist, R., Jukes, T. H., Moise, H., Goodman, M., and Moore, G. W., 1976. *J. Mol. Biol.* 105:39–74.
55. Moore, G. W., Goodman, M., Callahan, C., Holmquist, R., and Moise, H., 1976. *J. Mol. Biol.* 105:15–37.
56. Romero-Herrera, A. E., Lieska, N., and Nasser, S., 1979. *J. Mol. Evolu.* 14:259–266.
57. Romero-Herrera, A. E., Lehmann, H., Joysey, K. A., and Friday, A. E., 1973. *Nature* 246:389–395.
58. Romero-Herrera, A. E., Lehmann, H., Joysey, K. A., and Friday, A. E., 1976. In M. Goodman, R. E. Tashian, and J. H. Tashian (Eds.), *Molecular Anthropology,* Plenum Press, New York, pp. 289–300.
59. Romero-Herrera, A. E., Lehmann, H., Joysey, K. A., and Friday, A. E., 1978. *Phil. Trans. Roy. Soc.* 283:61–163.
60. Young, J. Z., 1962. *The Life of Vertebrates* (2nd ed.), Oxford University Press, New York.
61. Wilson, A. C., Carlson, S. S., and White, T. J., 1977. *Ann. Rev. Biochem.* 46:573–639.
62. Bakker, R. T., 1975. *Scientific American* (Apr.), pp. 58–78.
63. McLoughlin, J. C., 1979. *Archosauria,* Viking Press, New York.
64. McLoughlin, J. C., 1980. *Synapsida,* Viking Press, New York.
65. Fitch, W., 1970. *Syst. Zool.* 19:99–113.
66. Kimura, M., 1981. *J. Mol. Evolu.* 17:110–113 and 121–122.
67. Dr. Pangloss, 1759. In F. M. A. de Voltaire, *Candide.*
68. Kimura, M., 1968. *Nature* 217:624–626.
69. Kimura, M., 1979. *Scientific American* (Nov.), pp. 98–126.
70. King, J. L., and Jukes, T. H., 1969. *Science* 164:788–796.
71. Crow, J. F., and Kimura, M., 1970. *An Introduction to Population Genetics Theory,* Harper & Row, New York, Chapter 8.
72. Kimura, M., and Ohta, T., 1971. *Theoretical Aspects of Population Genetics,* Princeton University Press, Princeton, New Jersey.
73. Goodman, M., Tashian, R. E., and Tashian, J. H. (Eds.), 1976. *Molecular Anthropology,* Plenum Press, New York.
74. Johanson, D. C., and Edey, M. A., 1981. *Lucy: The Beginnings of Humankind,* Simon and Schuster, New York.

APPENDIX 3.1 MONOMERIC GLOBIN STRUCTURE ANALYSES[a]

Date	Protein	Source	Molecular weight	Amino acids	Analysis	References
1969	Hemoglobin, met, deoxy, oxy, CN⁻, CO	*Chironomus thummii*	15,410	136	1.4 Ref. 18% (oxy) and ΔF, ϕ_{met}	A1–A4
1971	Hemoglobin	*Petromyzon marinus*	16,566	146	2.0 MIR	A5, A6
1972	Hemoglobin	*Glycera dibranchiata*	15,595	147	2.5 MIR	A7, A8
1978	Leghemoglobin	*Lupinus luteus*	17,300	153	2.0 Ref.	A9, A10
1979	Leghemoglobin/nicotinic acid	*Lupinus luteus*	17,300	153	2.8 MIR	A11

[a]For explanation, see Appendix 2.1.

APPENDIX 3.1 REFERENCES

A1. Huber, R., Epp, O., and Formanek, H., 1969. *Naturwissenschaften* 56:362–367.

A2. Huber, R., Epp, O., and Formanek, H., 1970. *J. Mol. Biol.* 52:349–354.

A3. Weber, E., Steigemann, W., Jones, T. A., and Huber, R., 1978. *J. Mol. Biol.* 120:327–336.

A4. Steigemann, W., and Weber, E., 1978. *J. Mol. Biol.* 127:309–338.

A5. Hendrickson, W. A., and Love, W. E., 1971. *Nature New Biol.* 232:197–203.

A6. Hendrickson, W. A., Love, W. E., and Karle, J., 1973. *J. Mol. Biol.* 74:331–361.

A7. Love, W. E., Klock, P. A., Lattman, E. E., Padlan, E. A., Ward, K. B., Jr., and Hendrickson, W. A., 1972. *Cold Spring Harbor Symp. Quant. Biol.* 36:349–357.

A8. Padlan, E. A., and Love, W. E., 1974. *J. Biol. Chem.* 249:4067–4078.

A9. Vainshtein, B., Harutyunyan, E., Kuranova, I. P., Borisov, V. V., Sosfenov, N. I., Pavlovsky, A. G., Grebenko, A. I., and Nekrasov, Y. B., 1978. *Kristallografiya* 23:517–526.

A10. Vainshtein, B. K., 1981. *Struct. Stud. Mol. Biol. Interest* (G. Dodson, J. P. Glusker, and D. Sayre, Eds.), Oxford University Press, pp. 310–327.

A11. Harutyunyan, E. H., Tovlis, A. B., Crelenko, A. I., Voronova, A. A., Nekrasov, Yu. V., and Vainshtein, B. K., 1980. *Kristallografiya* 25:526.

APPENDIX 3.2 GLOBIN SEQUENCES AVAILABLE FOR EVOLUTIONARY COMPARISONS

As of the beginning of 1982, the authors could find complete and dependable amino acid sequences for 60 members of the α hemoglobin family, 66 from the β family, 60 myoglobins, and 11 monomeric globins.* These are listed by species in the table that follows, by the symbols:

α hemoglobin family: α = alpha chain; ζ = zeta (embryonic) chain

β hemoglobin family: β = beta chain; γ = gamma (fetal) chain; F = other fetal or immature, including tadpole; δ = delta chain; ε = epsilon (embryonic) chain

M = myoglobin, and G = monomeric globin chain

*See note at the end of Appendix 3.2 on page 115.

If several chains of a given type are present, they are identified by: α1, α2, or by letters: βA, βB, βC, etc.

All of the sequences in this appendix were compared in order to establish the invariant positions shown in Table 3.1 and in Figure 3.2. For the statistical comparisons leading to Table 3.5 and in Figure 3.15, only the sequences in boldface type were used. These were chosen in order to achieve a better illustrative balance among all phyla of vertebrates and invertebrates, since the total set is heavily weighted toward mammals. The sequence count and number of invariant residues can be summarized as follows:

Class of globins	Total number of sequences	Evolutionary invariant in:		Number used in Table 3.5
		Mammals only	All vertebrates	
α Hemoglobin family	60	50	23	32
β Hemoglobin family	66	51	20	35
Myoglobins	60	71	27	27

The principal source of amino acid sequence information is the *Atlas* of *Protein Sequence and Structure* (12), augmented by a February 1982 computer printout from the *Protein Sequence Database* provided by M.O. Dayhoff. A listing of 53 vertebrate myoglobin sequences provided by F. R. N. Gurd added several Cetaceans not yet entered into the *Database*.

Species	Globin sequence
PRIMATES	
Man *(Homo sapiens)*	**α** ζ / **β** γ δ ε / **M**
Chimpanzee *(Pan troglodytes)*	**α** α3 / **β** γ δ / M
Gorilla *(Gorilla gorilla beringei)*	**α** α3 / **β** δ / M
Gibbon *(Hylobates agilis)*	**β** δ / M
Olive baboon *(Papio anubis)*	α / **M**
Orangutan *(Pongo pygmæus pygmæus)*	M
Langur *(Presbytis entellus)*	**α** / **β**
Siamang *(Symphalangus syndactylus)*	M
Night monkey *(Aotus trivirgatus)*	**β** δ
Spider monkey *(Ateles geoffroyi)*	**α** / **β** δ
Capuchin monkey *(Cebus apella)*	**α** / **β**
Savannah monkey *(Certopithecus æthiops)*	**α** / **β**
Humbolt's wooley monkey *(Lagothrix lagothricha)*	M
Crab-eating monkey *(Macaca fascicularis)*	M
Japanese monkey *(Macaca fuscata)*	**α** / **β**
Pig-tailed macaque *(Macaca irus)*	**β** γ / M
Rhesus monkey *(Macaca mulatta)*	**α** / **β**
Squirrel monkey *(Saimiri sciureus)*	**β** δ / M
Tamarins *(Saguinus mystax)*	**β** δ
Common marmoset *(Callithrix jacchus)*	α / β / **M1** M2
Common tree shrew *(Tupaia glis balangeri)*	α / β / **M**
Bush baby *(Galago crassicaudatus)*	**M**
Potto *(Perodictius potto edwarsi)*	M
Sportive lemur *(Lepilemur mustelinus)*	α / β / **M**
Tarsier *(Tarsius bancanus)*	α / β
Slow loris *(Nycticebus coucang)*	**α** / **β** / **M**

LAGOMORPHS
  Rabbit *(Oryctolagus cuniculus)*   **α / β / M**
RODENTS
  Mouse *(Mus musculus)*   **α1 α2 / β1** β2
  Rat *(Rattus norvegicus)*   **α1 α2 / β**
  Yellow-cheeked vole *(Microtus xanthognathus)*   β
  Guinea pig *(Cavia porcellus)*   α / β
CHIROPTERIDS
  Fruit bat *(Rousettus ægyptiacus)*   M
CARNIVORES AND PINNIPEDS
  Dog *(Canis familiaris)*   **α1** α2 / **β / M**
  Coyote *(Canis latrans)*   α / β
  Bat-eared fox *(Otocyon megalotis)*   M
  Cape hunting dog *(Lycaon pictus)*   M
  Badger *(Meles meles)*   α / β / **M**
  Harbor seal *(Phoca vitulina)*   **M**
  California sea lion *(Zalophus californianus)*   **M**
CETACEANS
  Sperm whale *(Physeter catadon)*   **M**
  Dwarf sperm whale *(Kogia simus)*   M
  Minke whale *(Balænoptera acutorostrata)*   M
  Sei whale *(Balænoptera borealis)*   M
  Finback whale *(Balænoptera physalus)*   M
  California gray whale *(Eschrichtius gibbosus)*   **M**
  Pilot whale *(Globicephala melæna)*   M
  Humpback whale *(Megaptera novæangliæ)*   M
  Hubb's beaked whale *(Mesoplodon carlhubbsi)*   M
  Killer whale *(Orcinus orca)*   M
  Goose-beaked whale *(Ziphius cavirostris)*   M
  Common dolphin *(Delphinus delphis)*   M
  Amazon river dolphin *(Inia geoffrensis)*   **M**
  Pacific spotted dolphin *(Stenella attenuata graffamani)*   M
  Bottlenosed dolphin *(Tursiops truncatus)*   **M**
  Common porpoise *(Phocæna phocæna)*   **M**
  Dall porpoise *(Phocœnoides dalli dalli)*   M
PROBOSCIDEANS
  Indian elephant   M
PERISSODACTYLS
  Horse *(Equus caballus)*   **α1** α2 / **β / M**
  Donkey *(Equus asinus)*   α
  Zebra *(Equus burchelli)*   M
ARTIODACTYLS
  Cow *(Bos taurus)*   α / β **F / M**
  Sheep *(Ovis aries)*   α / β **βC** F / **M**
  Barbary sheep *(Ammotragus lervia)*   **α1 α2 / βC(NA)**
  Goat *(Capra sp.)*   **α1 α2 / βA** βC
  Llama *(Lama peruana)*   α / β
  European red deer *(Cervus elaphus)*   M
  White-tailed deer *(Odocoilus virginianus)*   **α1 α2**
  Pig *(Sus domestica)*   α / β / **M**
INSECTIVORES
  European hedgehog *(Erinaceus europæus)*   α / β / **M**

MARSUPIALS		
Oppossum *(Didelphis marsupialis)*	α / β / **M**	
Gray kangaroo *(Macropus giganteus)*	**α / β**	
Red kangaroo *(Megaleia rufa)*	β / **M**	
Potoroo *(Potorous tridactylus)*	β	
Echidna *(Tachyglossus aculeatus aculeatus)*	**α1 α2** / **β** / M	
MONOTREMES		
Platypus *(Ornithorhynchus anatinus)*	**α** / **β** / **M**	
BIRDS		
Chicken *(Gallus gallus)*	**α1** α2 Pi α$_{Str}$ / **β** / **M**	
Grelag goose *(Anser anser)*	α / β	
Ostrich *(Struthio camelus)*	α	
Penguin *(Aptenodytes patagonica)*	M	
REPTILES		
Alligator *(Diplocynodon)*	M	
Viper *(Viper aspis)*	**α**	
AMPHIBIA		
Bullfrog *(Rana catesbiana)*	αC α$_F$ / β β$_F$	
Frog *(Rana esculenta)*	**β**	
South African toad *(Xenopus)*	β	
Newt *(Taricha granulosa)*	**α**	
BONY FISH		
Carp *(Cyprinus carpio)*	α / β / M	
Desert sucker *(Catostomus clarkii)*	**α**	
ELASMOBRANCHII		
Port Jackson shark *(Heterodontus portusjacksoni)*	**α** / **β** / **M**	
AGNATHA		
Lamprey *(Lampetra fluviatilis)*	G	
Sea lamprey *(Petromyzon marinus)*	G	
MOLLUSCA		
Gastropod *(Aplysia limacina)*	G	
Gastropod *(Busycon canaliculatum)*	G	
INSECTA		
Midge *(Chironomus thummii)*	G, CTT–III	
Midge *(Chironomus thummii)*	G, CTT–II β	
ANNELIDA		
Bloodworm *(Glycera dibranchiata)*	G	
PLANTÆ: Leghemoglobins		
Soybean *(Glycine max)*	G	
Kidney bean *(Phascolus vulgaris)*	G	
Broad bean *(Vicia faba)*	G	
Lupine *(Lupinus luteus)*	G	

Note: On page 102 of their *Atlas* (Ref. 7, Ch. 2), Fermi and Perutz cite globin invariance results seemingly at odds with our conclusions. They report 27 invariant positions among 38 α chains, 18 invariants among 37 β chains, and only *nine* invariant positions among 55 myoglobins. The α and β discrepancies of 4 and 2 arise from the use of slightly different sets of sequences and are of no significance. But with myoglobin, the addition of gummy shark A and B chains deletes 5 invariants, and 14 more are eliminated by their inclusion, as myoglobins, of three invertebrate globins from the molluscs *Busycon, Aplysia kurodai,* and *Aplysia limacina.* The latter actually is to be found at the bottom of our Table 3.1 among the other invertebrate globins. These are myoglobins only in the general sense that the oxygen storage function of globin preceded that of oxygen transport. In any event, their inclusion would give a misleading impression of the variability of *vertebrate* myoglobins, for comparison with α and β hemoglobin chains. Using equivalent data sets, myoglobin appears slightly less variable than the hemoglobin chains.

Mutation map of human hemoglobin. Heavy circles indicate positions where altered amino acids have been observed in mutant human hemoglobins. Those mutations that lead to abnormal hemoglobin behavior are distinguished by solid color in the closest two subunits only, α_1 and β_2. More than 450 separate variants have been found at more than 170 of the 287 positions of human α and β chains. Mutations of all kinds are scattered at random over the entire hemoglobin molecule, but the pathological mutations tend to cluster around the heme pocket and the crucial $\alpha_1\beta_2$ sliding contact zone. The $\beta6$ location of the hemoglobin S or sickle-cell mutant is indicated at upper left and right by a black dot. A surface glutamate has been replaced by an uncharged valine. The reason why an apparently innocuous mutation on an out-of-the-way corner of the molecule should have such a catastrophic effect is a major topic of this chapter.

4 ABNORMAL HUMAN HEMOGLOBINS

CHAPTER 4

ABNORMAL HUMAN HEMOGLOBINS

When considering the delicately structured hemoglobin molecule, and the gene structure necessary to produce it, one can be forgiven for expressing amazement that such a complicated system should ever work. In fact, it frequently does not work, and that is the subject of this final chapter. By examining defective hemoglobins, considering how they are defective, and seeing what effect this has on the properties of the molecule, we can learn more about structure–function relationships than we possibly could from a simple examination of the normal hemoglobin. The properties of the abnormal hemoglobin H, with four β chains, and hemoglobin Bart's, with four γ chains, and the fact that the α chain cannot form a tetramer, will lead us at the end of the chapter to a possible reconstruction of the evolution of a functional hemoglobin tetramer.

Defects in the hemoglobin system that lead to anemia or other pathological symptoms are of three main kinds: breakdowns in transcription or processing of the messenger RNA needed to cause synthesis of the globin chains, point mutations in the DNA that lead to amino acid changes in the polypeptide chains, or outright deletions of sections of the globin genome (1, 2). Sickle-cell anemia is the classical point mutation disease, and will be considered later in the chapter. Other point mutations can lead to instabilities of the T or R state of the hemoglobin tetramer or both, or can interfere in other ways with normal globin function, but none is so serious (and so well studied) as the replacement of Glu $\beta6(A3)$ by Val in sickle-cell hemoglobin, also called *hemoglobin S*.

Regulatory failures or gene deletions that result in decreased or absent α or β globin chains are called α- and β-*thalassemias,* respectively (2–4). They are named from the Greek *thalassa* ("sea") because they are particularly common in areas surrounding the Mediterranean basin: Spain, Italy, Yugoslavia, Greece, Turkey, the Near East, and North Africa. Sickle-cell anemia is also common in this area. Heterozygous individuals (that is, people who have received an abnormal gene from one parent but a normal one from the other) are more resistant to malaria than normal individuals are, even when the hemoglobin defect is so serious that homozygotes having defective genes from both parents fail to survive (5). (Resistance to malaria is reasonably well documented for sickle-cell anemia, and less so but highly suggestive for thalassemia.) Thalassemias and sickle-cell anemia also are found in parts of southern China and Southeast Asia, India, and West and Central Africa—all regions where malaria is, or once was, common (Figure 4.1).

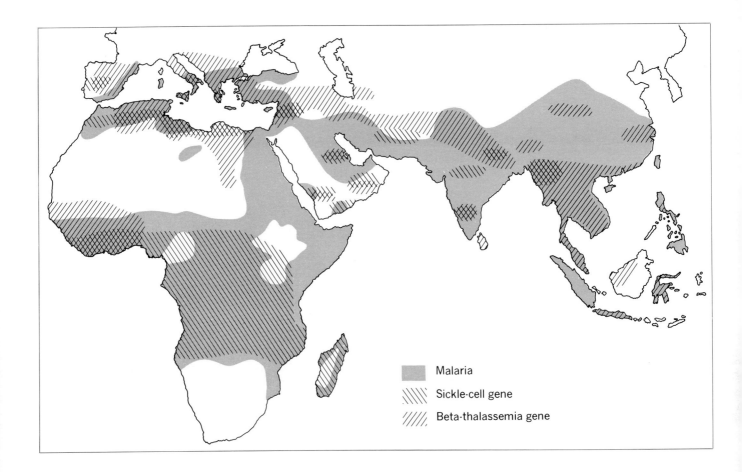

The special fitness of heterozygotes in comparison with either homozygotic form—two normal genes or two defective genes—is termed *overdominance*. The resultant carrying in the population of two genes, rather than the elimination of one or the other by natural selection, is an example of *balanced polymorphism*. At first glance overdominance is particularly surprising when one of the homozygotes represents the normal healthy individual and the other homozygotic state is lethal. Why should having one defective gene be better than having either two or none? We shall return later in this chapter to the molecular basis of malaria resistance in heterozygotes of these anemias (5). At the moment it is worth noting that this illustrates an important evolutionary principle: The thalassemia and sickle-cell defects survive in the human population *because* they confer a slight advantage to their heterozygous carriers. If this were not so, then the defects would slowly have been eliminated from the population by natural selection.

Figure 4.1 Correlation of malarial regions with hemoglobin diseases. Sickle-cell anemia and β-thalassemia are especially prevalent in those regions of the world where malaria was common before modern methods of eradication and treatment came into use. People who are heterozygous for either β-thalassemia or the sickle-cell gene have a slightly increased resistance to malaria for reasons that are described in the text. This amounts to a mechanism of survival for unfavorable genes that otherwise would be weeded out of the population by natural selection. Adapted by permission from Reference 5. Copyright by *Scientific American*, all rights reserved.

4.1 β-THALASSEMIAS AND β GENE DEFECTS

The term *β-thalassemia major* denotes the homozygous state with two defective genes, and *β-thalassemia minor* denotes the heterozygous state, with one normal and one defective gene. β-Thalassemia major results in severe anemia, and nearly always in death during childhood (1). The anemia does not arise simply from an undersupply of β chains for the tetramer. The unused α chains themselves cause trouble; they denature, precipitate onto the red blood cell membrane, damage the membrane and cause accelerated red cell destruction, resulting in hemolytic anemia. The cells are hypochromic, with a washed-out pallor arising from their low hemoglobin content, and frequently are misshapen. Bone marrow activity is overstimulated in a vain effort to counteract the hemoglobin shortage by producing more red blood cells, but most of these cells are destroyed before they reach the bloodstream. This hyperactivity of bone marrow can result in severe skeletal and cranial bone deformation. β-Thalassemia major, also known as *Cooley's anemia* after the person who studied and described it in North American populations in 1925, is the most serious of all thalassemias, being responsible for an estimated 100,000 child deaths per year (1).

In contrast to the foregoing bleak picture, the heterozygous or carrier state, β-thalassemia minor, can be accompanied by very mild symptoms or none at all. The red blood cells have a shorter average lifetime than in a normal individual, but this can be completely unimportant except under conditions of malnutrition or unusual stress (1). Unfortunately, these are exactly the conditions that exist today in large areas of sub-Saharan Africa where the defect is common.

Two types of β-thalassemia are known: β^+-thalassemia, in which the production of β chains is greatly reduced, and β^0-thalassemia, in which production is eliminated entirely. Both forms actually are groups of disorders, with common end results but multiple causes. β^+-Thalassemias generally involve processing defects at the mRNA stage, rather than outright deletion of β genes or defects in the regions that code for protein sequence (the exons). Too few β chains are synthesized because the messenger is present in inadequate amounts, but the chains that do result are normal. In some cases this seems to arise from mutations within the intervening sequences or introns of the β gene (Figure 3.7). These mutations, although they have no effect on the ultimate amino acid sequence, make it more difficult for the raw RNA as transcribed from the gene to be edited into a functional messenger for the ribosomes.

There are several causes for the total shutdown of β-chain production in β^0-thalassemias. Transcription or processing of the messenger may be blocked completely, so that no β-globin mRNA is produced. In other individuals, up to 30% of the normal level of messenger is produced, but no β-globin chains result; this has been traced to point mutational defects in the codon sequences. Examples are known where a nonsense or termination codon in the DNA causes the ribosome to halt synthesis of the chain before the entire β chain is completed. In one rare form of β^0-thalassemia the lack of β chains arises from a small deletion in the β gene itself, removing the third exon and some noncoding DNA to either side.

By far the most common gene-deletion disorders are δβ-thalassemia and hereditary persistence of fetal hemoglobin (HPFH). As with β^0-thalassemia, no β chains are produced at all by homozygous individuals. However, the usual almost complete shutdown of production of fetal γ chains in the normal adult is incomplete in these disorders, so an increase in $\alpha_2\gamma_2$ (hemoglobin F) can help make up the oxygen-carrying deficit. In δβ-thalassemia the marked increase in γ chains means that the homozygous state is relatively mild, and not as dangerous as β-thalassemia major. The patient has only hemoglobin F, but has enough to survive. In HPFH the production of γ chains appears to be totally unconstrained. Both heterozygous and homozygous HPFH individuals are known, and in general they are perfectly fit, with no clinical symptoms. HPFH and the δβ-thalassemias arise from large deletions of DNA sequence within chromosome 11 carrying the β family of genes (Figure 4.2).

Most deletions in the genome come about from unequal crossing-over during meiosis, produced by misalignment of the two chromosome chains just before crossover. Since misalignment is more likely if the DNA sequences being paired resemble one another, deletions frequently run from a given region in one gene to the analogous region in a closely related gene. A particularly clear example of this is a deletion mutant known as *hemoglobin Lepore*, which illustrates on a smaller scale the kind of deletions encountered in $\delta\beta$-thalassemia and HPFH. As Figure 4.2 shows, the deletion in hemoglobin Lepore is from one region in the β gene to the corresponding region in the δ gene. Figure 4.3 shows in more detail how this deletion occurs. The β gene on one chromosome is mispaired with the δ gene on the other. Crossover then results in two kinds of hybrid: one with only a single δ/β gene whose first part derives from the δ gene and whose second part comes from the β, and another chromosome with normal δ and β genes separated by a β/δ hybrid. These are termed *Lepore* and *Anti-Lepore*, respectively. The exact point of crossover in the hybrid gene varies from one individual to another. At least three different Lepore types have been encountered, termed *Boston, Baltimore,* and *Hollandia* after the places where they were found. There are also at least three different anti-Lepore types, more commonly known as *Miyada, P Congo,* and *P Nilotic.* (The letter *P* is a carryover from early days when it was thought that mutant hemoglobins could be identified by letters of the alphabet. Far too many mutants now are known, and current practice is to use geographical names denoting where the particular defect was first encountered. The term *hemoglobin M* still persists for those mutations that result in methemoglobin, in which the iron is oxidized rather than oxygenated.)

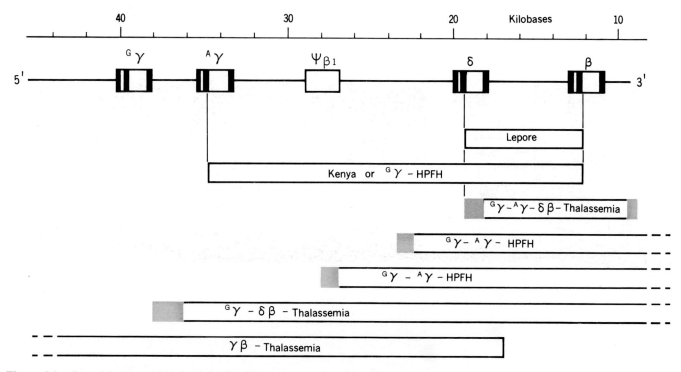

Figure 4.2 Gene deletions within the β family. The genes are taken from Figure 3.7, with their relative positions measured in thousands of bases from the 3′ end shown above. Bars below indicate regions that are deleted in various disorders. Shaded regions indicate uncertainties in the beginning or end of a deleted region. (Adapted from Reference 2.)

Individuals heterozygous for hemoglobin Lepore, having one normal and one Lepore hybrid chromosome, produce roughly half the normal quantity of hemoglobin A, and 10–15% as much hemoglobin Lepore tetramer having two α chains and two hybrid δ/β. The ratio is not 50:50 because the hybrid gene is not expressed as well as the normal β. In compensation, slightly more hemoglobin F is produced, and the mild anemia that results can be totally harmless. In contrast, the homozygous Lepore state found in a few individuals is more serious; no hemoglobins A or A₂ at all, and only a moderate amount of Lepore tetramer. The victim survives only because of an overproduction of fetal hemoglobin F. Hemoglobin Lepore is a model example of a clearly understood gene-deficiency disease. In its inverse, anti-Lepore, the individuals have one or both chromosomes with normal δ and β genes as well as the β/δ hybrid (Figure 4.3). Such individuals function normally because they have the complete set of hemoglobin genes, and the presence of the extra hybrid β/δ gene ordinarily is detected only during blood testing for some other purpose.

Of the more extensive HPFH deletions, hemoglobin Kenya ($^G\gamma$-HPFH) has a deletion extending all the way from the β gene at the right to the equivalent region of the $^A\gamma$ fetal gene at the left (Figure 4.2). In the other cases diagrammed in the figure, the exact location of the ends of the deletion is not as well known, but the missing regions have been characterized. $^G\gamma$-$^A\gamma$-δβ-Thalassemia is so named because, although both the δ and β chains have been deleted, both of the fetal genes $^G\gamma$ and $^A\gamma$ are intact and expressed, albeit at a low level. Some region of chromosome 11 to the left of the δ gene must play a part in turning off the fetal genes in a normal human adult, since deletion of this region leads to

Figure 4.3 Mechanism of deletion by crossover of mismatched DNA. If two genes have a general resemblance in sequence, and if their flanking sequences (vertical shading) to either side also are similar, then the DNA strands can become misaligned during meiosis. Crossover then results in hybrid genes. For δ and β genes, the consequence is three genes on one chain after crossover and one on the other. In hemoglobin Lepore heterozygotes, the individual had one normal two-gene chromosome and one chromosome with a single δ/β hybrid gene, and in heterozygous hemoglobin anti-Lepore a normal pair of genes is combined with a three-gene strand. Observations of the amino acid sequences in the hybrid chains provide evidence for the order of δ and β genes along the chromosomes.

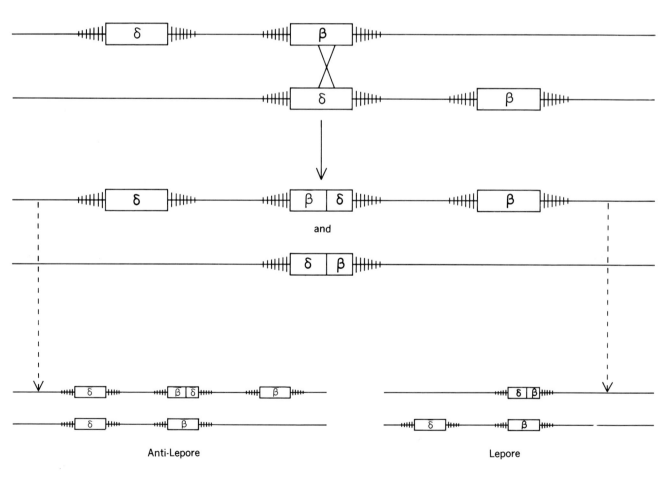

Anti-Lepore

Lepore

$^{G}\gamma$-$^{A}\gamma$-HPFH, in which enough fetal chains are made to compensate fully for the loss of δ and β. Two different forms of this HPFH have been found, differing by the extent of the deletion at the left end. Extending the deletion at the left nearly to the $^{G}\gamma$ gene, so that the $^{A}\gamma$ gene is deleted, lowers the overall production of γ chains to the point where a $\delta\beta$-thalassemia, known as $^{G}\gamma$-$\delta\beta$-thalassemia, is the result. Two examples of total $\gamma\beta$-thalassemia are known, in which the defective chromosome makes none of the β family of chains. This disorder obviously has been encountered only in heterozygous individuals, where a second normal copy of the chromosome is available to provide the β chains necessary to keep the victim alive. A curious aspect of $\gamma\beta$-thalassemia is that the β gene is present and intact, although not used. The suggestion has been made that both genes of a pair, δ and β, or $^{G}\gamma$ and $^{A}\gamma$, are required for either one to be expressed properly, and this may be one aspect of gene control. In $\gamma\beta$-thalassemia, the absence of the δ gene is presumed to suppress β synthesis. The ability to clone and study large amounts of genetic material means that we can expect to learn much more about gene control and expression in the next few years.

4.2   α-THALASSEMIAS AND HEMOGLOBIN HOMOTETRAMERS

In contrast to the defects in the β-producing chromosomes, most of the α-thalassemias appear to be simple gene-deletion diseases, arising from the loss of one, two, three, or all four of the α genes possessed by normal individuals on their two copies of chromosome 16. The main clinical problem is anemia from the shortage of α chains, since these are needed for every kind of functional tetramer other than the embryonic Gower-I ($\zeta_2\varepsilon_2$) and Portland ($\zeta_2\gamma_2$). The excess γ and β chains form homotetramers: hemoglobin Bart's (γ_4) and hemoglobin H (β_4). Both of these bind oxygen tightly, as in the R state of normal hemoglobin, show no R-to-T transition, fail to release oxygen cooperatively at low partial pressures, and lack a Bohr effect. The x-ray analysis of hemoglobin H has shown that the molecule indeed has the R or oxy configuration (6) (see Figure 2.16). In contrast, no α_4 tetramers are formed in any of the β-thalassemias; the α chains seem to be unable to hold together. The main structural difference between α and β subunits is the absence of a D helix in the former, and this suggests some ideas about the structural requirements for a functional tetramer, which will be considered again in Section 4.5.

The β chains have a greater attraction for α chains in tetramers than γ chains have (1), so when both β and γ chains are present along with an inadequate supply of α, hemoglobin A ($\alpha_2\beta_2$) forms in preference to F ($\alpha_2\gamma_2$), relegating the leftover γ chains to hemoglobin Bart's (γ_4). Only when the amount of β chain by itself is greater than that of α will appreciable hemoglobin H (β_4) be observed.

Four grades or degrees of clinical severity are known for α-thalassemia, and these can be equated with the loss of increasing numbers of the four α hemoglobin genes (Figure 4.4):

1. *The silent-carrier state (α-thalassemia 2)*. One gene is missing. This condition is entirely symptomless. About 1–2% hemoglobin Bart's is present at birth, from leftover γ chains.

2. *Classical α-thalassemia trait (α-thalassemia 1)*. Two genes are missing. About 5% hemoglobin Bart's is present at birth. Minor red blood cell abnormalities occur later, but no anemia or other symptoms. As Figure 4.4 indicates, individuals with this grade could either be homozygotes with one α gene per

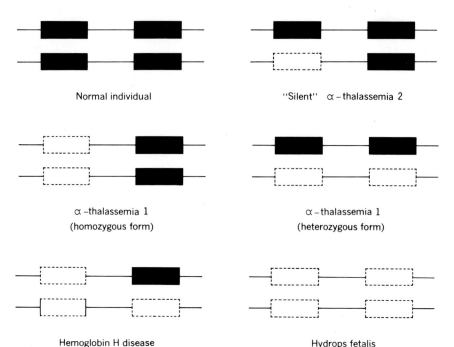

Figure 4.4 α-Gene deletions in various types of α-thalassemia. Genes present are represented by dark boxes, and deleted genes by dotted outlines. Each normal individual has two copies of chromosome 16, each bearing two adjacent genes for α hemoglobin chains. Deletion of increasing numbers of genes leads to diseases of increasing clinical severity. α-Thalassemia 1 with two deleted genes can occur in homozygous and heterozygous forms, which can be distinguished genetically even though their symptoms are equivalent. (Adapted from Reference 2.)

Normal individual

"Silent" α – thalassemia 2

α –thalassemia 1
(homozygous form)

α –thalassemia 1
(heterozygous form)

Hemoglobin H disease

Hydrops fetalis

chromosome, or heterozygotes with two genes on one chromosome and none on the other. They can be distinguished genetically even though the clinical symptoms are the same. Asian α-thalassemia 1 patients tend to be heterozygous, whereas Mediterraneans and African blacks usually are homozygous.

3. *Hemoglobin H disease.* Three genes are missing. Anemia is intermediate between that of β-thalassemia minor and major. Hemoglobin Bart's is present from the excess of γ chains in infancy, and hemoglobin H is present in the adult.

4. *Hydrops fetalis.* All four α genes are missing. This is invariably fatal, leading to stillbirth in the last few weeks of pregnancy, presumably because the supply of ζ chains is no longer sufficient to keep the fetus alive via hemoglobins Gower-I and Portland. Interestingly enough, just as deletion of the δ and β genes can remove the controls damping down the synthesis of γ chains in HPFH, so the deletion of both α genes causes the ζ gene to continue to be expressed long after it would have been shut down during embryonic development. The compensation is not, however, enough to keep the fetus alive until birth. These represent two examples of a cluster of genes also possessing a control region able to shut down a more distant group of genes when they are no longer needed.

One of the most common types of α-thalassemia leading to hemoglobin H disease and *hydrops fetalis* in the Orient is interesting in that it involves having too much of a good thing, rather than a deletion. In hemoglobin Constant Spring, the TAA ochre termination codon at what should be the end of an α gene has mutated to CAA, which is the codon for glutamine. Hence the RNA polymerase blithely continues reading past the end of the normal gene, and adds the codons for 31 extra amino acids before it encounters another stop codon. In the α chain that results, amino acids Tyr 140 and Arg 141 are followed by Gln 142 and a tail of 30 more amino acids. This extra tail makes the chains unusable in forming $\alpha_2\beta_2$ tetramers, and the same effect is produced as if the α gene had simply been deleted. Approximately 20% of the observed hemoglobin H patients have the hemoglobin Constant Spring defect.

The thalassemias tell us much about hemoglobin gene structure, but less about hemoglobin molecular structure, aside from the clues about evolution of the tetramer that will be discussed later. But hemoglobin S, sickle-cell hemoglobin, is the best studied of a number of disorders that arise from point mutations and single changes in amino acid sequence. These are useful in pointing out the critical and the less essential regions of the hemoglobin molecule. They can serve as a check on the structure–function proposals that were made in Chapter 2 from the examination of normal hemoglobins.

Sickle-cell anemia is the classic example of a genetic hemoglobin disease (1). Many of the techniques that later were used to study and analyze the thalassemias were first tried out with sickle-cell anemia. Before the origin of either the sickling or the anemia was known, it was nevertheless clear that the malady was transmitted in a classical Mendelian manner. Two levels of severity were encountered: the quite severe sickle-cell anemia proper, and the almost symptomless sickle-cell trait. These were shown in 1949 to be the homozygous and the heterozygous carrier states of the same unknown genetic defect. As with the thalassemias, the defect is especially common in regions where malaria is present, because it gives increased malarial resistance to heterozygotes (Figure 4.1). In North America it is therefore especially prevalent among the black population of African descent.

The most striking aspect of the disease, and the source of its name, is the tendency for red blood cells to adopt a contorted banana or sickle shape at low oxygen concentrations (Figure 4.5). The blood of a person with sickle-cell anemia behaves more or less normally at the 100-mm Hg oxygen pressure at the

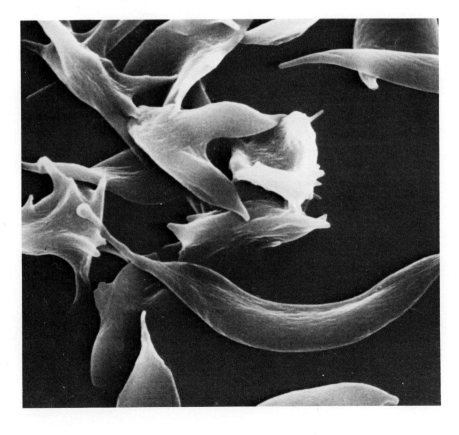

Figure 4.5   Scanning electron micrograph of sickled erythrocytes. Normal red cells are biconcave discs (Figure 2.1), whereas sickled cells are contorted by the presence of aggregations of hemoglobin fibers within the cell, and often assume long crescent shapes. Photo courtesy of W. N. Jensen, Albany (N. Y.) Medical College.

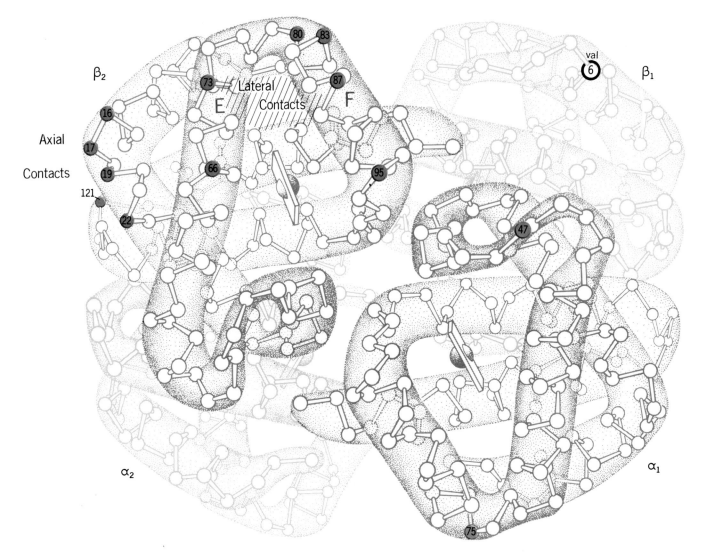

Figure 4.6 Intermolecular contacts in sickled fibers. Residues in color have been identified as contacts from hybrid mutant studies. Residues 66, 73, 80, 83, and 87 of one β subunit form an acceptor pocket that interacts with a mutant β6 valine from an adjoining molecule. These are termed the *lateral contacts*. (See discussion on page 133, and Figures 4.16 and 4.19.) Contacts along the fiber direction are termed *axial contacts* and include residues 16, 17, 19, 22, and 121. Other positions, including β95, α47 and α75, are believed to be involved in contacts between twisted filaments of the sickled fibers. Residues β85 and β88, although crucial to the lateral contacts, are not revealed by mutant studies because they are so essential that altering them incapacitates the molecule. Data from R. M. Bookchin and R. L. Nagel.

lungs, aside from some long-term damage to erythrocyte membranes caused by previous bouts of sickling. However, at the lower oxygen pressure at which hemoglobin delivers its O_2 in the tissues (40 mm Hg), there is a tendency for the cells to adopt the distorted shape. These cells, deformed and more rigid than normal erythrocytes, are trapped in the capillaries, causing pain and inflammation. Even where outright sickling does not occur, the aggregation and polymerization of deoxyhemoglobin S molecules inside the erythrocytes makes them stiffer and less able to bend and slip flexibly through the microcirculation system as they should. Most sickled cells regain their normal shape when reoxygenated, but a certain number of them suffer membrane damage and become irreversibly sickled cells (ISCs). These defective cells are fragile and have a shorter than average lifetime, making the patient anemic and placing a heavy load on the erythrocyte-generating machinery of the bone marrow. Homozygous individuals can survive to adulthood if given adequate levels of nutrition, health care, and protection from stress, particularly infection and hypoxia. But in the more stringent conditions of the African Congo, the widespread existence of sickle-cell anemia actually was missed by investigators for many years because homozygous children usually died before they reached the age at which they would have been routinely screened by health workers (1).

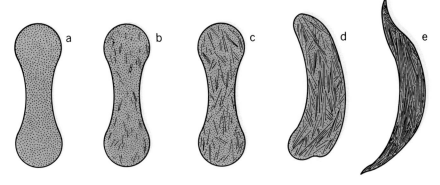

In contrast to homozygotes, heterozygous carriers of the sickle-cell trait usually show no symptoms at all. Sickling does not occur to an appreciable extent unless the oxygen pressure sinks to 25 mm Hg or less, and this happens only under unusual circumstances such as high-altitude flying in unpressurized aircraft, some severe forms of pneumonia, or inadvertent anoxia during anesthesia.

Linus Pauling proposed in 1949 that sickling arose from a defect in the hemoglobin molecules, and he coined the term *molecular disease* (7). He suggested that these defective molecules might aggregate into bundles of rods upon deoxygenation, and thereby twist the erythrocytes out of shape. Seven years later Vernon Ingram showed precisely what this defect was: The sixth amino acid along each β chain in the hemoglobin tetramer is not glutamic acid as in a normal chain, but valine (8). A negatively charged side chain is replaced by a hydrophobic one. When the three-dimensional structure of hemoglobin was deciphered in 1960, one could see that the altered side chain sat at position A3 in the first alpha helix of each β subunit, exposed at corners of the tetramer (Figure 4.6). Such an altered molecule is termed hemoglobin S. But why should a change in only two of the 574 amino acids of a hemoglobin molecule produce such a drastic effect as sickling?

The historical background of the long effort to understand the sickling phenomenon has been described in several excellent reviews (9–11). In brief, the concentration of hemoglobin molecules in red blood cells is so high (340 mg/mL) that they almost could be said to be on the verge of crystallization even under normal conditions. The $\alpha_2\beta_2$ tetramers, spheroids of axial dimensions 65 by 55 by 50 Å, are only 10 Å apart on the average, so it is surprising that they can rotate and flow past one another without hindrance. Anything that would make them more "sticky" might be expected to increase the viscosity of the solution, lower the solubility of the molecules, and cause them to aggregate. This, indeed, is what seems to be accomplished by replacement of a negative charge at position β6(A3) on the surface by an "oily" or hydrophobic residue. When deoxygenated, the defective hemoglobin S molecules aggregate in a specific manner to form long fibers, and these group themselves into bundles of columns that stiffen the cell and push it into an elongated sickle shape. Figure 4.7 illustrates how the fiber formation could distort the cell shape. It also illustrates how the mechanical properties and flexibility of the erythrocyte can be adversely affected by sickle-fiber formation even before the deformation of the cell membrane becomes obvious. Schechter and Noguchi have used NMR spectroscopy to detect polymers of deoxyhemoglobin S molecules in sickle-cell erythrocytes at relatively high oxygen saturation values. This raises the possibility that these cells are not behaving normally, even on the arterial side of the microcirculation (11).

Figure 4.7 Progressive formation of fibers, and deformation of the cell membrane during sickling. Bundles of oriented, sickled fibers form within the erythrocyte and, when sufficiently extensive, begin to deform the cell membrane. However, the fiber domains can cause trouble by making the erythrocytes less flexible and less able to traverse the capillaries, even before the onset of visible sickle deformation of the cell envelope. From left to right the separate illustrations represent oxygen saturation values of: (a) 100%, (b) 75%, (c) 50%, (d) 25%, and (e) 0%. Adapted by permission from Reference 11.

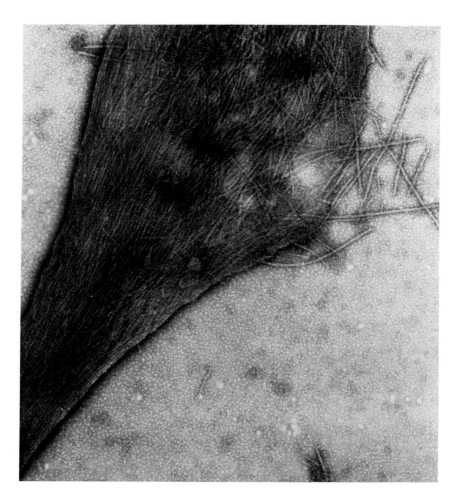

Figure 4.8 Sickled fibers from a burst erythrocyte. Electron micrograph of fibers of deoxyhemoglobin S spilling out of a ruptured cell. Individual fibers are approximately 220 Å in diameter, and in some a helical twist pattern can be seen. (From Reference 14.)

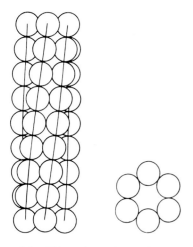

Figure 4.9 Side and top views of the first model of the helical 180 Å sickled fiber, consisting of stacks of 6-membered rings of sickled deoxyhemoglobin tetramers. This now is considered to be a rare polymeric form of hemoglobin S. (From Reference 10.)

Murayama proposed in 1966 that deoxygenated hemoglobin S molecules stack spontaneously into sixfold helical rods or columns, and that the oily patch produced by Val 6 might be in a particularly favorable position to cause interaction with neighboring molecules in the deoxygenated state, but not the oxy (12, 13). Murayama's stacking interactions were wrong in detail; he proposed that the Val β6 interacted with Val β1 in the same subunit, and that the true twofold axis of the hemoglobin tetramer (vertical in Figure 4.6) lay along the fiber axis, whereas we now know that it is perpendicular to the axis. But the work represents a pioneering attempt to explain why hemoglobin S forms fibers and causes sickling in the deoxy state but not the oxy.

Figure 4.8 shows a dramatic view of a sickled cell whose outer membrane has been disrupted by hypotonic lysis—placing the cells in low-salt solution so they burst like sausage casings (14). The sickled fibers are clearly visible, spilling out of the cell into solution at the right. Within the cell, the fibers are packed more or less in parallel along the long axis of the distended erythrocyte. Electron micrographs of thin sections through the sickled cell, or of stained preparations of packed, centrifuged fibers after release from the cell, reveal two kinds of filaments: 180 Å diameter strands, with cross-spacings perpendicular to the filament axis every 64 Å (suggestively close to the horizontal dimension of the tetramer in Figure 4.6), and 200–240 Å diameter strands whose cross-striations appear to be at an angle to the filament axis (15, 16). The thin fibers are not often seen, and were interpreted by Finch et al. as six-stranded, twisted cables (15) as in Figure 4.9.

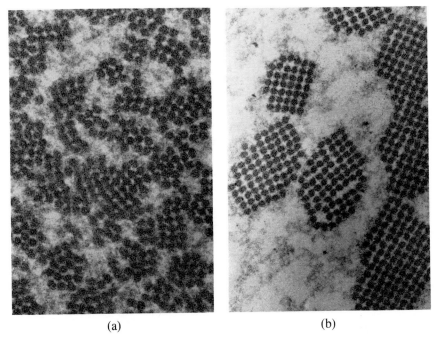

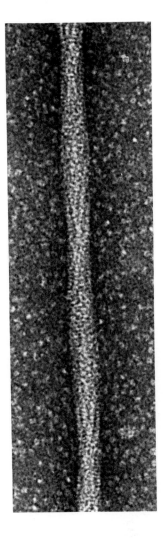

Figure 4.10 Cross sections of bundles of 220 Å fibers. (a) Fibers obtained directly from a sickled cell, with packed center-to-center distances of 217 ± 11 Å. (b) Fibers reconstituted by stirring a solution of deoxyhemoglobin S, with center-to-center distances of 214 ± 9 Å, essentially identical to (a). (From Reference 18.)

Figure 4.11 Transverse view of a twisted fiber and its molecular interpretation. The variable diameter of the fibers and their twisted appearance suggest a helical fiber with noncircular cross section, as in the electron micrograph at left. The model at right is made up from four inner strands of hemoglobin tetramers (circles), surrounded by another outer layer of ten strands, all given a right-handed helical twist with a periodicity of 3000 Å per complete turn. The outer ten strands have been removed in the middle of the drawing to show the packing of the four-strand core. (From Reference 21.)

Josephs, Edelstein, and their respective co-workers, while not ignoring the thin filaments, consider the more ubiquitous 220 Å strands to be more significant (16–23). An 8-strand model was initially proposed for these strands, but this, like the 6-strand models, has been abandoned in favor of more complex structures. At present the field is divided into protagonists of the 14-strand model proposed by Edelstein and co-workers (17–21), and protagonists of the 16-strand model put forth by Josephs and colleagues (22–25). Each model has compelling arguments in its favor. There is no way for an outside observer to adjudicate an issue on which even the professionals are in such disagreement, and we shall not even try. Few of the really important molecular or medical issues, however, stand or fall on the choice of one model over the other as being correct.

Cross sections through bundles of the 220 Å diameter fibers in the sickled cell show that the fibers are packed in square or hexagonal arrays with an average of 220 Å between centers (Figure 4.10a). Even more highly ordered arrays can be produced by first oxygenating the solution so the hemoglobin S is dissolved, and then stirring the solution gently under deoxygenating conditions, which causes sickle fibers to form (Figure 4.10b). The fibers are not perfectly cylindrical. They seem to have an oval or elliptical cross section that, combined with a slow twist in the fiber axis, gives the filament a varying width and a helical appearance, as in Figure 4.11. Three-dimensional image reconstruction methods using electron micrographs have led to the 14-strand model that is shown in a cutaway fiber drawing in Figure 4.11, and in cross section in Figure 4.13. This model can be described as a close-packed core of 4 strands, surrounded by an outer envelope of 10 strands, also in close-packed array. These 14 strands seem to be associated in seven pairs. Occasional micrographs of incomplete 10-strand and 6-strand fibers suggest that they might arise from the 14-strand model by loss of pairs as shown by the gray outline in Figure 4.12, and therefore also suggest a particular pattern of pairing of strands in the complete fiber.

The alternative 16-strand model is best approached after a discussion of the single-crystal x-ray structure analysis of hemoglobin S. Wishner, Love, and co-workers crystallized the protein directly from solution and solved its structure to 3 Å resolution (A1, A2). Tetramer molecules in the deoxyhemoglobin S crystals are packed against one another in zigzag double strands, as in Figure 4.14. One Val β6 from each tetramer is packed against an "oily" or hydrophobic depression in a tetramer from the other strand, just as would be expected if these chains of tetramers in the crystal were related to sickled fibers in solution. Adjacent zigzag chains in the crystal are antiparallel; they run in opposite directions as in Figure 4.14. Equal numbers of chains running in each direction are packed together within the crystal in the manner shown in the top view of Figure 4.15.

The single-crystal analysis of hemoglobin S showed the molecular structure and intermolecular packing in great detail, much more than could ever be learned by electron microscopy and x-ray analysis of sickle fibers. But it was not clear at first whether the intermolecular contacts in the crystal were at all relevant to the contacts between molecules in sickled fibers. Then Magdoff-Fairchild made the dramatic discovery in 1979 (26) that sickled fibers sealed in glass capillaries for

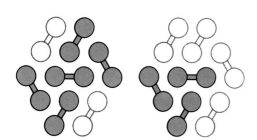

Figure 4.12 Ten-strand and 6-strand sickled fibers (color) occasionally are seen that look as if they were obtained from a 14-strand fiber by loss of the particular pairs of fibers shown here in gray outline. This limits the way in which the strands can be paired in the intact fiber. (From Reference 19.)

Figure 4.13 Computer reconstuction of fiber cross section. This is a computer-generated image of a cross section through the 14-strand fiber model depicted in Figure 4.11, obtained by analysis of electron micrographs. Each peak represents one strand of hemoglobin tetramers running perpendicular to the page. (From Reference 19.)

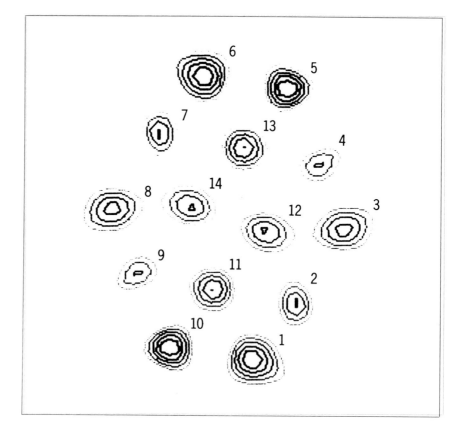

x-ray study slowly converted over several years to crystals that apparently were identical in x-ray pattern to those freshly grown from solution and analyzed by Love. Pumphrey and Steinhardt had discovered earlier that needlelike crystals could be obtained from hemoglobin S solutions by stirring (27, 28), and Wellems and Josephs continued this approach by showing that when highly purified hemoglobin S solutions are stirred for several hours, thin fibers first develop and collect into bundles or fascicles, and these fascicles then anneal to form true crystalline needles and twisted ribbons (14, 22, 23). The connection between crystal structure and sickle-fiber structure must be very close.

This close relationship between fibers and crystals led Josephs and Wellems to propose their 16-strand model for the sickled fibers. It essentially is a fragment of the crystal structure, composed of 8 zigzag double strands as in Figure 4.15—4 running in one direction and 4 in the opposite direction. It has the advantage of equal numbers of antiparallel strands; the 14-strand model, if composed of 7 double strands, could at best have 4 such double strands running one way and 3 the other. Annealing 14-strand fibers into a Wishner–Love crystal would require bringing in isolated double strands to fill in the chinks, an aesthetically unsatisfying although not impossible procedure.

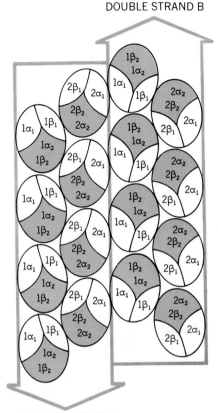

Figure 4.14 Antiparallel double strands of hemoglobin S. In this view, looking down the *c* axis of the hemoglobin S crystal, zigzag double strands of tetramers (here labeled double strands A and B) are packed against one another in antiparallel fashion. In this view, subunits α_1 and β_1 are side by side at one end of each tetramer, and subunits α_2 and β_2 are superimposed at the other end. If this latter end is considered as the "front" of the molecule, then this figure shows the way in which double strands A and B run in opposite directions.

Figure 4.15 Packing of double strands in deoxyhemoglobin S crystals. In this top view down the *a* axis of the crystal, the four double strands labeled B run toward the viewer with their α_2 and β_2 subunits nearest, whereas the four double strands A below run downward into the page.

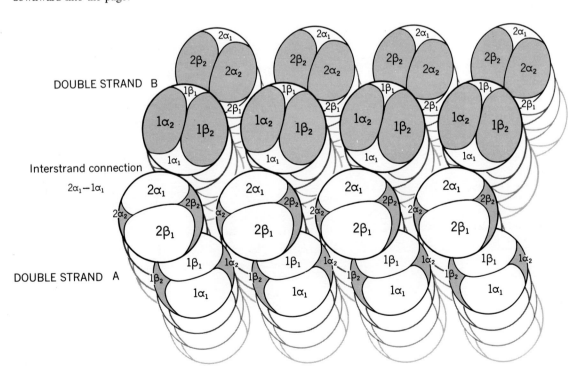

The arrangement of molecules in the double strands of crystalline hemoglobin S is shown schematically in Figure 4.16 below, and in detail in the stereo pair on the opposite page (Figure 4.18). This work revealed for the first time just why the presence of valine at position β6 leads to sickling. Valine from a tetramer in one strand fits into a hydrophobic pocket at the EF corner in a

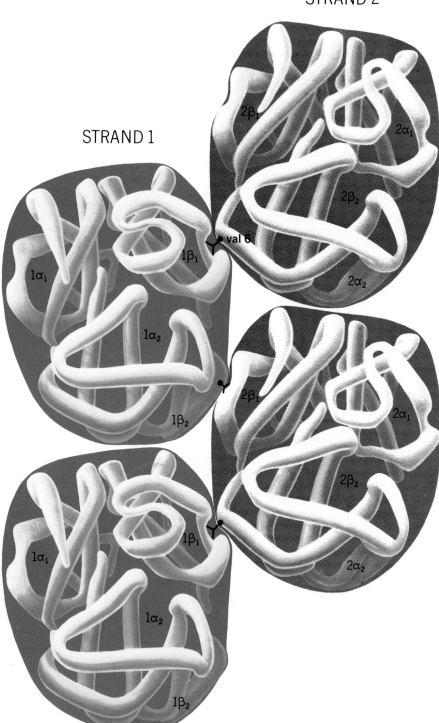

Figure 4.16 Close-up of the deoxyhemoglobin S double strand. This view is the same as that of strand A in Figure 4.14, with the α₂ and β₂ subunits superimposed at the bottom of each molecule, and the α₁ and β₂ subunits side by side at the top. The hidden portions of overlapped molecules are not shown. Lateral contacts between strands involve Val β6 as donor and the EF pocket of a molecule on the adjoining strand as acceptor. Axial contacts connect molecules vertically along the same strand. Hemes have been omitted for clarity but are shown in the stereo drawing (Figure 4.18) from which this figure was derived. Details of lateral and axial contacts are shown in Figure 4.20, and the interacting surfaces involving the mutant β6 are shown in Figure 4.24.

tetramer from the other strand. That molecule, in turn, fits a Val β6 from its *other* β chain into a hydrophobic EF pocket in the next molecule up or down the chain in the original strand. The result, in what must be considered an example of cosmic bad luck, is that molecules that show no tendency to stick together when glutamic acid occurs at β6 now adhere into a long fiber, and a molecular disease is born.

The critical Val β6 and the hydrophobic EF pocket are marked on the hemoglobin drawing of Figure 4.6. They occur on different β chains; each tetramer contributes only one connecting valine and one hydrophobic acceptor pocket. It has been possible to map out the important parts of the molecule using naturally occurring mutant hemoglobins having a single amino acid change, of the type that will be considered in the next section. If a mutant has a change in an α chain, then a hybrid molecule can be made in solution using these α chains and the β chains from hemoglobin S (29). Beta-chain hybrids also can be prepared, in which one of the β chains is the test mutant and the other comes from hemoglobin S (30, 31). It is more difficult to find mutant hemoglobins that have a second amino acid change on the β chain that bears the Val β6(A3), but a few are known. These hybrid test molecules then can be studied to see if they are any less prone, or more prone, to form gels than is hemoglobin S. (Gel formation in the test tube is analogous to fiber aggregation in the red blood cells.) If a difference in solubility behavior is observed, then the changed amino acid presumably lies in a region of intermolecular contact in sickle fibers. If no change in solubility results, the situation is less definite; either the region is not a sickle contact, or the altered amino acid is as acceptable at the contact zone as the normal one.

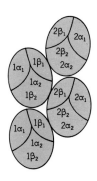

Figure 4.17 Scheme of subunit assembly in the hemoglobin S double strand.

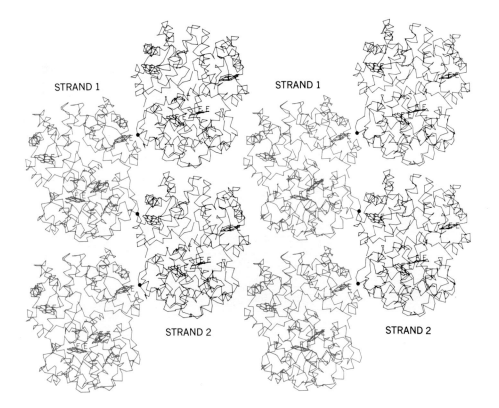

STRAND 1

STRAND 1

STRAND 2

STRAND 2

Figure 4.18 Computer-generated stereo pair drawing of deoxyhemoglobin S double strands, from the crystal-structure analysis. Strand 1 is in color and strand 2 is in black. Main chains are depicted schematically by straight lines connecting α-carbon positions, which occur at bends. The Val β6 positions that are involved as donors in fiber formation are marked by black dots, and hemes are labeled FE. (Computer drawing from R. Feldmann, NIH, based on crystal structure coordinates from W. Love, Johns Hopkins.)

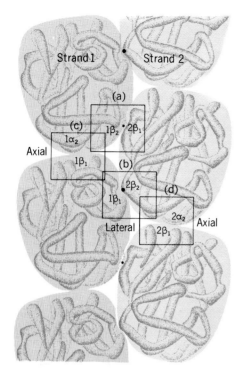

Figure 4.19 Location of lateral and axial contacts in the double strand of the deoxyhemoglobin S crystal. Details of contacts are shown below in Figure 4.20.

The results of these solubility experiments are mapped onto the hemoglobin molecule in Figure 4.6. Around the acceptor pocket, altering side chains β73, 80, 83, or 87 decreases the tendency toward gel formation, whereas changing Lys 66 to Glu enhances gelation. On the left side of the molecule lies a region that is termed the *axial contact* because it is the contact between molecules within a given strand, along the fiber direction. Changing residues 16, 17, 19, or 22 decreases gelation, whereas altering Glu 121 to Gln or Lys increases it. The last two mutations are also known to increase the severity of sickle disorders in individuals heterozygous for one of these mutations and for hemoglobin S. The Gln 121 mutation is known as hemoglobin D Los Angeles or D Punjab, and the Lys 121 mutation is called hemoglobin O Arab.

These solution studies are confirmed and extended by the intermolecular contacts seen in the single-crystal analysis, reinforcing the proposal that crystals and sickle fibers are very similar in their arrangement of hemoglobin tetramers. The two rows of tetramers in the crystalline double strand (Figure 4.19) are related only by an approximate screw symmetry operation; the axial contacts in strand 1 are similar but not identical to those in strand 2, and the lateral contacts between Val β6 in strand 1 and an acceptor pocket in strand 2 again are similar but not identical to those between the strand 2 valine and the strand 1 acceptor pocket. These four regions of intermolecular contact are shown in more detail in Figure 4.20a–d. In all of these drawings, the subunit donating the Val β6 to the lateral contact is labeled β2, and that supplying the acceptor pocket is β1. Strand numbers, 1 or 2, precede the α or β. Hence 2β2 signifies the β subunit on strand 2 that contributes a valine to the contact with subunit 1β1 on the other strand. Figure 4.20a and b confirm the involvement of Lys 66, Asp 73, Asn 80, Gly 83, and most especially Thr 87 in the lateral contacts, and adds Gly 69, Ala 70, His

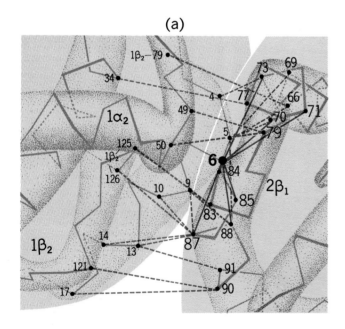

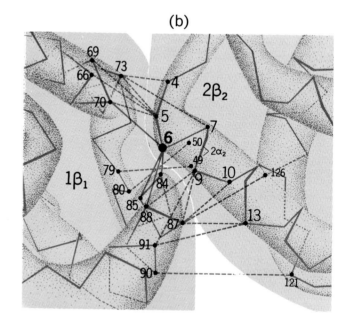

Figure 4.20 (a and b) Side chain packing contacts of 5 Å or less between molecules in a hemoglobin S double strand, as determined by the x-ray crystal structure analysis. Contacts involving Val β6 are colored solid lines; other contacts are dashed. (a) Lateral contacts between donor subunit 1β2 and acceptor 2β1. (b) Lateral contacts between donor 2β2 and acceptor 1β1. These are chemically similar but not crystallographically identical in the x-ray study.

77, Asp 79, Thr 84, Phe 85, Leu 88, Glu 90, and Leu 91 to the list. On subunit β_2, Val 6 is not the only side chain involved in the contact. Others to either side are also involved, as are even Ser 49 and His 50 on the adjacent CD corner of an α subunit. In Figure 4.20c and d, Gly 16, Lys 17, Asn 19, Glu 22, and Glu 121 are involved, as the mutant hemoglobin studies suggest, but many others of their immediate neighbors in the axial contacts at the AB and GH corners of the β and α subunits are also.

The preceding comparisons are strong and compelling evidence that the contacts between tetramers within a zigzag double strand are the same in the crystal and in sickled fibers. But what about the contacts between different double strands? These almost certainly will not be the same; the double strands are packed linearly in the crystal, whereas they are twisted in the sickle fibers (Figures 4.21, 4.22). Crystal-like contacts at one point in the fiber could be turned out of registration farther along the helix. As Figure 4.21 indicates, in the crystal the contacts between double strands involve mainly the α chains, including His 45, Phe 46, and Asp 47 at the CD corner; Ala 53, Gln 54, Lys 61, and Asn 68 in the E helix; His 72, Asp 75, Asn 78, and Ala 79 at the EF corner; and Leu 80, Ser 81, and Ala 82 in the F helix. Edelstein has attempted to calculate the contacts that would be expected in a twisted helical 14-strand fiber, and these predictions can be tested as a means of evaluating the 14-strand model (32). Lys β95 does not appear to be a contact point in the crystal structure, although it is exposed prominently on the front face of the molecule. But since replacing Lys β95 by either Asn or Glu reduces the gelation tendency of solutions of hybrid hemoglobin S molecules, this location must be of some importance in sickling, and seems to represent a true difference between crystal and fiber.

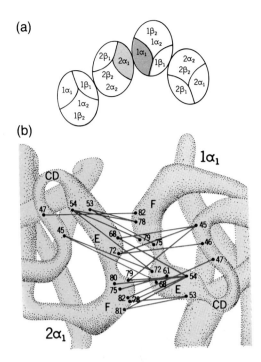

Figure 4.21 (a) Location of contact regions between antiparallel double strands in the crystal. (b) Scheme of contacts beween subunits $2\alpha_1$ and $1\alpha_1$ in different antiparallel strands.

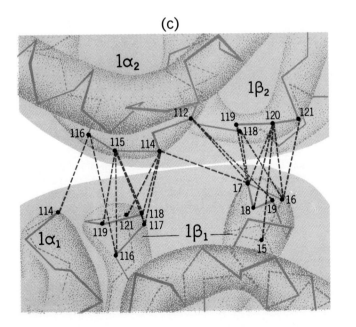
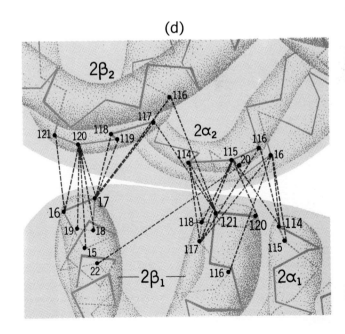

Figure 4.20 (c and d) Axial contacts between tetramers in the same strand, 1 or 2, along the strand axis. This corresponds to the fiber direction in sickle-cell fibers. (c) Contacts involving A helices and GH regions along strand 1. (d) Similar contacts along strand 2. In a–d, the path of the main chain is represented by straight black lines, with α-carbon positions at bends. Contact data are from Appendix 4.2; 1981 coordinates from E. Padlan and W. Love.

Figure 4.22 Twisting of the double strand as is observed in sickled fibers. In fibers, unlike crystals, the double strands are twisted into a right-handed helix. Contacts between molecules within one such twisted double strand probably resemble those in the crystal, but the contacts between double strands could be quite different from those in the untwisted double strands of the crystal.

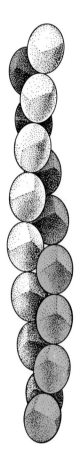

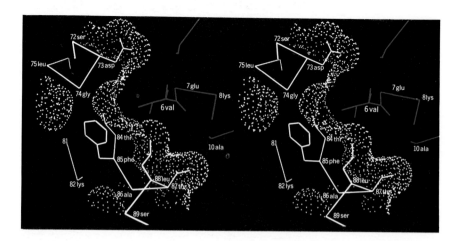

Figure 4.23 Computer-generated stereo pair drawing of the EF acceptor pocket at the lateral contact in deoxyhemoglobin S, with Val β6 from the donor in place. Main chain is represented by straight lines, white for the EF acceptor corner and color for the Val β6 donor. The molecular surface of the acceptor is mapped out by white dots. Phe 85 and Leu 88 form the floor of the pocket, whose walls include Asp 73, Thr 84, and Thr 87. (See also Figure 4.25 at right.)

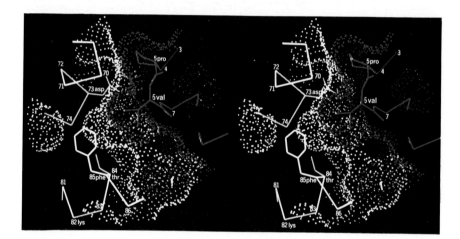

Figure 4.24 Fitting between donor (color) and acceptor molecules (white). The protrusions and hollows in the two molecular surfaces are remarkably complementary, which explains the tighter binding and the propensity for sickling in hemoglobin S with Val β6, compared with hemoglobin G Makassar, which has Ala at the same position and does not cause sickling. (Stereos produced at Scripps Clinic, La Jolla, in collaboration with Olson and Connolly, from refined deoxyhemoglobin coordinates of Love and Padlan.)

The key to sickling behavior is a hydrophobic acceptor pocket between the E and F helices that is present in deoxyhemoglobin but absent in oxyhemoglobin. The acceptor pocket is lined at the bottom with the side chains of Phe 85 and Leu 88, and has Asp 73, Thr 84, and Thr 87 around the perimeter. The actual fitting of Val β6 from another subunit into the pocket is shown in computer-generated stereo pair drawings in Figures 4.23 and 4.24. Helix A of the donor subunit begins at Thr 4 and Pro 5, and the critical Glu versus Val 6 is located in the first helical turn, followed by two other charged residues: Glu 7 and Lys 8. This cluster of two negative charges and one positive charge in normal hemoglobin A

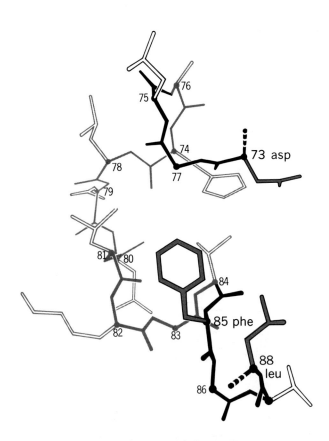

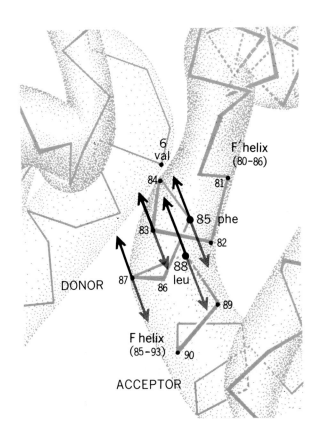

Figure 4.25 Main chain pathway of the EF acceptor pocket, in approximately the same viewing direction as the two previous stereos. Side chains Asp β73, Phe β85, and Leu β88, which interact with the donor, are shown in color. This is a view out through the EF corner from the interior of the molecule. The E helix runs from right to left across the top of the drawing, sinking into the page as it does so. The chain bends down and back at the left, and returns to the right with the F′ and F helix segments, rising toward the viewer in the process. Phe β85, closest to the viewer, actually sits at the very bottom of the acceptor pocket.

Figure 4.26 Motion of the F helix upon oxygenation and deoxygenation, in the lateral contact region as seen in Figure 4.20(a). Colored arrows indicate the shift toward the FG corner upon oxygenation, and black arrows show the F helix motion upon deoxygenation. The result of this motion is to make the side chains of Phe β85 and Leu β88 accessible to the surface in deoxy but not oxy, creating an acceptor pocket into which a Val β6 can fit. Walder and Arnone have shown that crosslinking the β82 lysines simulates the motion of the F helix in the deoxy to oxy transition as described on page 144 and in reference 46.

means that the beginning of the helix has no attraction for the hydrophobic EF pocket. But if residue 6 is changed from Glu to Val, then its side chain can nest snugly into the pocket in the manner depicted in Figure 4.24. The area of van der Waals contact is increased by packing Pro 5 against Gly 69 and Ala 70, and Ala 10 against Thr 87. (Contacts are detailed in Appendix 4.2.)

The critical Phe 85 that defines the floor of the acceptor pocket occurs just at the bend between the two parts of the F helix: F′ (residues 80–86) and F (residues 85–93). The motion of the F helix toward the FG corner upon oxygenation pulls Phe 85 toward the center of the molecule, away from potential contact with the sickling Val 6 side chain (Figure 4.26). Upon deoxygenation, the F helix motion brings Phe 85 back again and restores the hydrophobic pocket. Hence only in the deoxyhemoglobin conformation (or the T state) is the acceptor pocket shaped in a way that promotes interaction with hydrophobic side chains from the donor molecule, and only for this state does sickling occur.

AGGREGATION HIERARCHIES IN DEOXYHEMOGLOBIN S MOLECULES

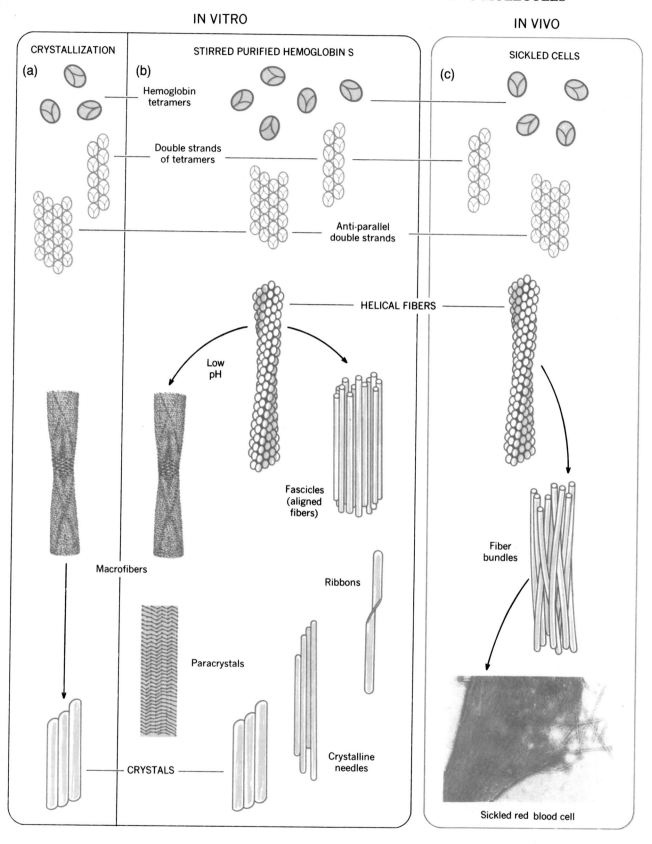

IN VITRO

IN VIVO

CRYSTALLIZATION

STIRRED PURIFIED HEMOGLOBIN S

SICKLED CELLS

(a)

(b)

(c)

Hemoglobin tetramers

Double strands of tetramers

Anti-parallel double strands

HELICAL FIBERS

Low pH

Fascicles (aligned fibers)

Macrofibers

Fiber bundles

Ribbons

Paracrystals

Crystalline needles

CRYSTALS

Sickled red blood cell

The connection between the known deoxyhemoglobin S crystal structure and sickled fibers has been made even more direct by experiments in the growing of gels from solution. Gels are ordered networks of fibers, of bundles of fibers, and ultimately of crystals themselves. The gelation and sickling phenomenon can be regarded as one of relative solubilities: Under physiological conditions, deoxyhemoglobin S has a solubility of only 160 g/L, whereas oxyhemoglobin S and both states of normal hemoglobin have solubilities in excess of 500 g/L (11). The solubility of deoxyhemoglobin S also is greater at 0°C than at room or body temperature. Eaton and Hofrichter have found that, when a solution of deoxyhemoglobin S is warmed rapidly from 0°C to 25°C, a considerable delay time ensues before it sets into a gel of ordered fibers (34–37). The delay time is inversely proportional to a large power of hemoglobin concentration, ranging from 15 to 30 in different experiments. This suggests that nuclei consisting of 15–30 hemoglobin molecules must form by a slower process before rapid fiber growth can take place. As has been mentioned, Pumphrey and Steinhardt discovered that, if the solution is stirred continuously during this latent period, crystals are the result rather than a gel (27, 28). The solution retains its fluidity, but contains bundles of needlelike crystals easily visible under a microscope. Apparently the shearing forces from stirring are sufficient to keep the growing fibers aligned well enough that they eventually coalesce into true crystals rather than an interlaced fiber network. Wellems and Josephs have studied the solution-to-fiber-to-crystal process in detail by electron microscopy (14, 22, 23), and their findings are summarized in Figure 4.27. The first visible change, when solutions of chromatographically pure hemoglobin S are warmed to 23°C with stirring, is the appearance of fibers. Optical diffraction patterns produced from electron micrographs indicate that these fibers are effectively identical to those obtained directly by lysis of sickled erythrocytes (Figure 4.8). Within 20 minutes, these fibers begin aggregating into loose bundles or fascicles with their long axes aligned (Figure 4.28). The alignment process within these fascicles continues more slowly. After approximately 5 hours of stirring, flat, ribbonlike crystals can be seen (Figure 4.29). In their early stages they seem to be helical ribbons, which flatten against the electron microscope grid like twisted paper strips, but they eventually grow into needles of appreciable thickness. By the eighth hour, conversion of the hemoglobin S solution to crystals is complete. Some molecular detail actually can be seen in electron micrographs of these crystals, and the observed repeat distances in the micrographs, 64 by 180 by 50 Å, match the crystalline unit cell dimensions. Hence it seems clear that sickled fibers can coalesce into crystals, closely related or identical to those studied by Wishner and Love, without major alteration other than perhaps an unwinding of the sickled strands so they might pack against one another in crystalline fashion. The helical twist observed in the first thin, ribbonlike crystals may in fact reflect a residual twisting that is being annealed out of the fibers as they crystallize.

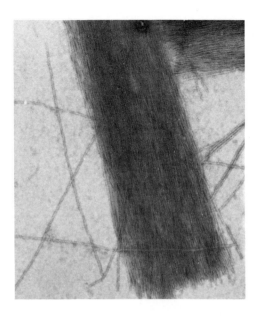

Figure 4.28 Electron micrograph of fascicles of hemoglobin S fibers obtained from a stirred solution. Although the fibers are aligned, they still have discrete boundaries and have not merged into one crystal. (From Reference 34.)

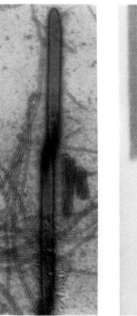
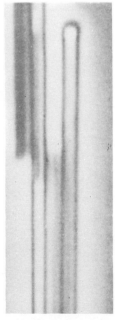

Figure 4.29 Micrographs of thin, twisted ribbons (left) that presumably already possessed a helical twist before being flattened onto the microscope grid, and (right) the larger crystals into which they grow with time. See top of page 141 for close-up of the twisted ribbon. (From References 14 and 22.)

Figure 4.27 Aggregation hierarchies in deoxyhemoglobin S molecules. (a) Crystallization directly from solution probably involves the aggregation of antiparallel double strands into macrofibers and the buildup of crystalline order from these. (b) In stirred hemolysates, tetramers first aggregate into fibers composed of antiparallel double strands, by a process whose details are not known. Fibers aggregate to form crystals by one of two pH-dependent pathways: annealing of bundles or fascicles of many aligned fibers, or growth of larger macrofibers that then transform into crystals. (c) In sickled cells the bundles of fibers presumably never achieve the lateral degree of order that permits them to crystallize, and hence the fibers remain as rods within the sickled cell.

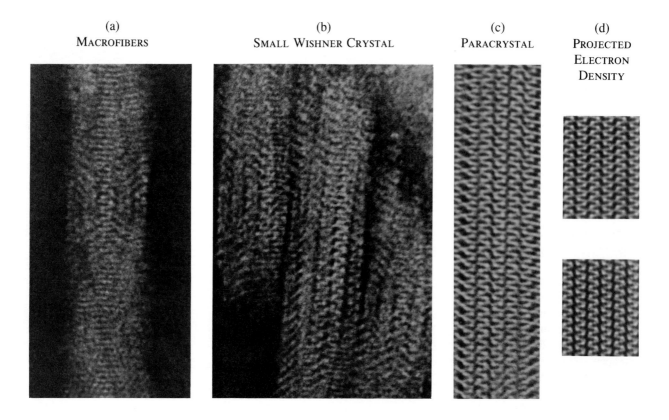

| (a) | (b) | (c) | (d) |
| MACROFIBERS | SMALL WISHNER CRYSTAL | PARACRYSTAL | PROJECTED ELECTRON DENSITY |

Figure 4.30 Fret and herringbone patterns in deoxyhemoglobin S assemblies. (a) Macrofibers grown from stirred purified deoxyhemoglobin. Note the appearance, near the center, of being constructed from several twisted cables. Note also the fret pattern of double strands and the herringbone pattern from aligned pairs of antiparallel double strands. (b) Small crystals grown as for the x-ray structure analysis. Note the similarity in herringbone pattern to macrofibers. (c) Well-ordered region from a paracrystal, revealing the herringbone pattern to arise from alignment of adjacent zigzag columns of molecules. (d) Calculated density patterns using the known crystal structure of deoxyhemoglobin S. Each vertical zigzag column is a double strand of tetramers. (Courtesy Robert Josephs.)

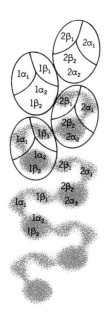

Figure 4.31(a) Molecular interpretation of zigzag double strands seen in Figure 4.30 as a fret pattern. The bright spots in the electron micrograph above are the regions where α_2 and β_2 subunits overlap when viewed down the c axis of the crystal.

The sequence of events just described is what is observed around pH 7 or above. At slightly lower pH, around 6, a different set of intermediate forms leads to the same final crystals, and this is the "low pH" pathway of Figure 4.27. Instead of forming large bundles that slowly anneal into crystals, the fibers grow first into larger macrofibers that already begin to show signs of crystalline order (Figure 4.30a). These increase in internal order still further to form paracrystals (Figure 4.30c), and finally true crystallinity is achieved. Paracrystals appear to be made up of well-ordered layers of double strands, but with misalignment or misregistration between layers. The final stage of crystal formation by this route is the sliding of double-strand sheets over one another into proper registration.

Figure 4.30b shows an electron micrograph of small hemoglobin S crystals of the type grown directly from solution for x-ray analysis. The similarity of pattern to macrofibers and paracrystals is apparent. Wellems, Vassar, and Josephs used the known atomic coordinates of hemoglobin S crystals to calculate what the antiparallel chains of double strands of tetramers in the crystals should look like at a resolution comparable with that of the electron micrographs, and the results are in Figure 4.30d. Each vertical zigzag chain is one double strand, and the distribution of larger white blobs (areas from which stain is excluded by protein) even show that adjacent chains run in opposite directions. This same antiparallel chain packing is visible in paracrystals (Figure 4.30c). The origin of the larger blobs of density is apparent from Figure 4.31: The superposition of α_2 and β_2 subunits in this projection excludes more stain from this part of the specimen, and brightens the image of the chain at that point. Figure 4.31a shows the origin of the fret pattern in a double strand, and Figure 4.31b shows the herringbone pattern when antiparallel double strands are aligned. This is an example of the way in which macromolecular structure information can be extracted from electron micrographs, if one can learn to "think like an electron beam" and interpret them properly.

In sum, the molecular mechanism by which a defect in a single amino acid in the β chain of hemoglobin leads to sickling of erythrocytes is now known in considerable detail. But does this suggest any way of ameliorating, controlling, or even preventing sickle-cell anemia? The most naive response would be, "Find something that gets in the way of the Val $\beta6$–acceptor pocket interaction and prevents sickle-fiber formation." But there are two troublesome problems: that of specificity, and that of delivery to the erythrocytes. Chemical reagents that modify hemoglobin S in a way that prevents sickling, but also modify many other proteins of the body, can be dangerous or lethal. Moreover, a successful therapeutic agent must be something that can be delivered to the interior of erythrocytes in the bloodstream of the patient. An ideal agent would be one that passes easily through the erythrocyte membrane, and interacts specifically and solely with hemoglobin, leaving other body proteins untouched or at least unharmed. No such wonder drug has yet been found.

It may not actually be necessary to prevent sickling outright; only to delay the onset of sickling for long enough after deoxygenation to permit the red blood cells to pass through the capillaries and into the larger venous system on the way back to the lungs (34, 37). Because of the very high 15–30th power dependence of gelation-delay time on hemoglobin concentration, a 10% decrease in de-oxyhemoglobin S concentration could increase the delay time by a factor of 10 or 100. Hence a potential therapeutic agent could be valuable even if it only delayed sickling, rather than preventing it. A 2% increase in erythrocyte volume would dilute deoxyhemoglobin S enough to double the delay time.

How much of a delay in the onset of sickling would be required to produce a significant therapeutic effect? This question has been addressed directly by examining heterozygous patients who have one hemoglobin S gene and either normal hemoglobin A, HPFH, or β^+-thalassemia at the other gene (37). (These will be identified as S/A, S/HPFH, and S/β^+, respectively.) In comparison with homozygous sickle-cell (S/S) patients, S/β^+ patients have a somewhat less severe anemia. The small amount of normal β chain that they produce dilutes their hemoglobin S enough to produce delay times 10 to 100 times as great. In comparison, S/HPFH patients have delay times 10^3 to 10^4 times as long as S/S homozygotes, and their anemia is much less severe, verging on the tolerable though inconvenient level. Most fortunate of all is the S/A heterozygote with sickle-cell trait. Such people have delay times greater than S/S by a factor of 10^6 or so. They show virtually no symptoms, and achievement of this level of amelioration in an S/S patient would justifiably be termed a cure. Hence the delay-time approach can be considered promising if a substance delays the onset of gelation in vitro by a factor of 10^4 to 10^6, and if the substance is such that it can be introduced into the erythrocytes without serious side effects elsewhere in the patient. These, as we shall see, are stringent and so far unfilled requirements.

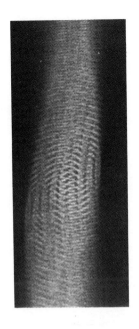

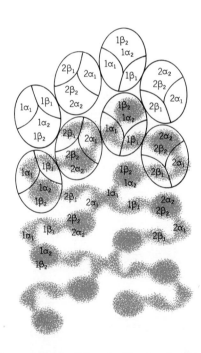

Figure 4.31(b) When double strands align as in Figure 4.30 they form a herringbone pattern, as schematized in the drawing above. At the top of the page is a closeup of a twisted ribbon from Figure 4.29, showing the herringbone pattern clearly.

TABLE 4.1 STRATEGIES FOR SICKLE-CELL THERAPY[a,b,c]

I. INTERFERENCE WITH SICKLING CONTACTS
  A. Noncovalent reagents
    1. Alteration of solution conditions
      a. Urea or guanidine hydrochloride to disrupt hydrophobic interactions
      b. Alkyl ureas
      c. Organic solvents, ethanol, detergents
    2. Stereospecific inhibitors
      a. Aromatic amino acids (phenylalanine, etc.) and peptides containing them
      b. Aromatic alcohols and acids
      c. Synthetic peptides mimicking β-subunit amino terminus or EF corner
    3. Gases (propane, ethane, dichloromethane)
  B. Covalent reagents
    1. Monofunctional reagents
      a. Cyanate carbamylation of amino terminus (extracorporeal administration because of peripheral nerve damage):
        i. α chain (predominant reaction)—favors R state ($>O_2$)
        ii. β chain (lesser reaction)—interferes with T-state tetramer contacts?
      b. Pyridoxal sulfate modification of α amino terminus—inhibits sickling ($=O_2$)
      c. Glyceraldehyde Schiff base modification of lysines—inhibits sickling ($=O_2$)
      d. Nitrogen mustard modification of His β82—interferes with sickling contact site, but too toxic; analogs under study
    2. Cross-linking reagents
      a. Dimethyl adipimidate (but unspecific cross-linking of many proteins, hence extracorporeal administration only)
      b. Bis (3,5-dibromosalicyl) fumarate—specific binding in DPG site, holds EF corners away from favorable sickling geometry
      c. Methylacetimidate—inhibits sickling ($=O_2$)

II. DECREASE IN DEOXYHEMOGLOBIN S CONCENTRATION
  A. Shift of equilibrium toward oxyhemoglobin S state ($>O_2$)
    1. Carbamylation or acetylation
      a. Cyanate—toxic side effects
      b. Carbamyl phosphate—may be less toxic
      c. Acetylation with dibromoacetylsalicylic acid
    2. Schiff-base adducts that specifically increase O_2 affinity and inhibit sickling: pyridoxal, 5-deoxypyridoxal, salicylaldehyde, o-vanillin
    3. Sulfhydryl modification at Cys β93 to stabilize R state
      a. Cystamine
      b. Bis (N-maleimidomethyl) ether—cross-links Cys β93 and His β97, shifts O_2 binding curve to left without loss of heme–heme cooperativity
    4. Adjustment to alkaline pH
  B. Increase in volume of erythrocytes
    1. Induced hyponatremia, swelling (but danger of water intoxication)
    2. Other agents that affect erythrocyte membrane permeability
  C. Induction of hemoglobin F overproduction by derepressing fetal γ genes
  D. Artificial insertion of normal β genes to induce hemoglobin A production

III. MODIFICATION OF ERYTHROCYTE MEMBRANE TO DIMINISH SICKLING TENDENCY
  Procaine hydrochloride, zinc acetate, Cetiedil, other experimental agents; little progress yet

IV. INHIBITION OF MICROVASCULAR ENTRAPMENT OF SICKLED CELLS
  Interesting future approach, not yet tested

---

[a]Adapted from reference 10.

[b]At present this table is much more a "shopping list" or statement of desired goals, rather than a catalog of successful treatments. There is no cure for sickle-cell anemia at present, only a collection of promising research approaches and partial therapies.

[c]($=O_2$), no change in oxygen affinity; ($>O_2$), increased oxygen affinity.

A "wish list" of chemotherapeutic approaches that have been tried, or which seem sensible to try, is given in Table 4.1. The most successful efforts so far (and no trials have been successful enough to yield what could remotely be termed a cure) are listed under I and II: interference with the sickling-fiber contacts, or dilution of the concentration of deoxyhemoglobin S. Experiments to modify the cell membrane have been inconclusive, and modifying the microvascular system to allow fewer sickled cells to be trapped is only a clever idea at present.

As soon as the nature of the contact between Val 6 and the hydrophobic EF pocket became known, one obvious therapeutic approach was to attempt to disrupt hydrophobic contacts in general, or this specific contact in particular. Nonspecific "chaotropic" or disordering agents such as detergents, ethanol, and other organic solvents were of little value; their contribution to dissolving hemoglobin S gels in vitro was counterbalanced by their random effect on other macromolecules, and their toxicity in vivo. It is easy to find agents that disrupt gels in vitro, and thus have therapeutic potential. It is quite another matter to find ways of administering the substance to patients so that it is delivered to sickled erythrocytes in high enough concentration to be useful without exhibiting toxic side effects. Two potential candidates, urea and cyanate, foundered on these difficulties in the early 1970s. Urea looked interesting because it is known to disrupt hydrophobic interactions. Yet careful double-blind clinical studies conducted by the National Institutes of Health with intravenously administered urea showed it to have no measurable effect at tolerable dosage levels (10, 38). In the laboratory, it increased the delay time for the onset of gelation by only a factor of 2, much too low to suggest therapeutic value.

Some of the other substances that have been considered as antisickling agents are shown in Figure 4.32. Alkyl ureas (urea derivatives with hydrocarbon side chains) seemed promising from gelation studies, but the toxicity problem has not been solved. Cyanate ion is a breakdown product of urea in aqueous solution, and once was thought to be the active agent in urea treatment. However, it does more than simply disturb hydrophobic contacts between molecules. It specifically carbamylates the free amino groups at the α-chain amino termini, and to a lesser extent those on the β subunits and on lysine side chains. This amino-terminus modification destabilizes the T state of the hemoglobin tetramer relative to the R state, as we saw in Chapter 2, and hence increases the oxygen affinity, decreasing the concentration of the molecular form that is capable of sickling. But once again, clinical tests showed no practical therapeutic effect, and there was evidence of peripheral nerve damage to the patients (10). Gelation-delay times of 6- to 30-fold at the 1 or 2 millimolar concentration level are still far too low to be useful. Oral administration of sodium cyanate has been abandoned, but some consideration is still being given to extracorporeal cyanate treatment of blood.

An interesting "molecular engineering" approach is to design short peptides that adopt conformations in solution mimicking the offending Val β6 chain, the EF acceptor pocket, or one of the intermolecular fiber contacts (39, 40). Hydrophobic amino acids such as phenylalanine are marginally effective, increasing the solubility of deoxyhemoglobin S by 8–12%, but phenylalanine has toxic side effects in children. Short peptides containing phenylalanine are no more effective than the amino acid itself, and longer peptides actually make deoxyhemoglobin S *less* soluble because they tie up water molecules. However, a decapeptide containing the amino acid sequence of residues 82–91 of the β chain (the EF corner) does actually inhibit gel formation. It may be promising as a "molecular cuckoo," wrapping itself around Val β6 and preventing it from participating in sickle-fiber contacts.

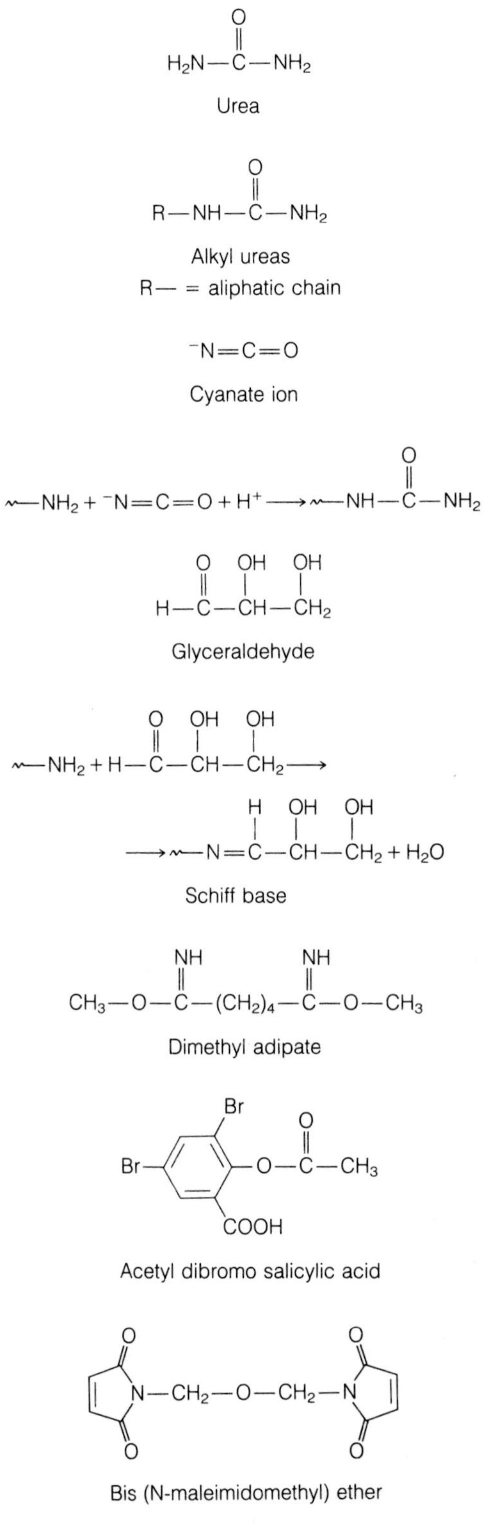

Figure 4.32 Chemical reagents that have been considered in sickle-cell chemotherapy experiments. They range from small molecules such as urea that simply destabilize proteins, to specific cross-linking agents.

Figure 4.33 Bifunctional reagents for crosslinking lysine side chains. Efficiency of crosslinking depends critically on the length and geometry of the connecting chain. Bromine atoms facilitate entry through the erythrocyte membrane.

Bis (3,5-dibromosalicyl) esters:

fumarate:

succinate:

general case:

Crosslinking:

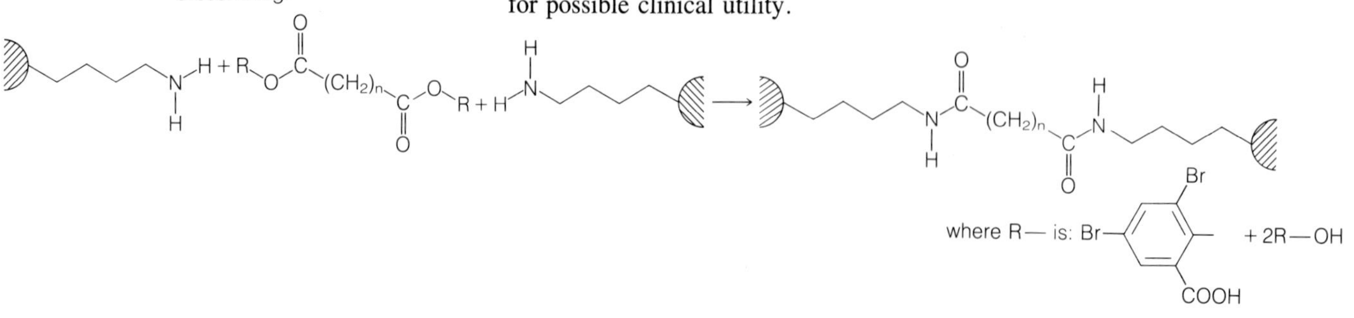

An alternative to blocking the sickle-fiber contact sites would be to keep more of the tetramer in the R state, in which it has the wrong geometry for building sickle fibers. This is the mode of action of cyanate and other reagents that modify the α amino termini. Substances such as glyceraldehyde (41), imidates including dimethyl adipimidate (42), and acetyldibromosalicylic acid (43) react with amine groups and decrease gel formation in vitro, and the last "bromoaspirin" approach may offer real clinical possibilities. The acetylsalicylates are particularly gentle acylating reagents for lysines and amino termini, and adding nonpolar groups such as halogen atoms around the salicylic acid ring improves the ease with which the drugs can slip through the erythrocyte membrane (44).

Specific cross-linking reagents have been used to hold the molecule in the R conformation. Bis(N-maleimidomethyl) ether (Figure 4.32) cross-links Cys β93 to His β97 on the same subunit and shifts the oxygen-binding curve (Figure 2.5) to the left, decreasing the proportion of deoxyhemoglobin S at any given O_2 partial pressure. Another group of bifunctional reagents, bis(3,5-dibromosalicyl) esters of fumaric, succinic, and other dicarboxylic acids (Figure 4.33) are even more specific in their action (44–46). They occupy the DPG site in the tetramer, cross-linking two Lys β82 side chains on the two β subunits in the R state, as depicted in Figure 4.34. The dibromosalicyl compounds are more effective than those without bromines, in part because they can pass through the erythrocyte membrane more easily. The length of the chain is critical for cross-linking; 4-carbon connecting chain molecules (with $n = 2$) in Figure 4.33 (succinate derivatives) are most effective whereas longer chains are less so. Recent solubility studies by Walder (47) show that succinate increases solubility by 50% over native deoxyhemoglobin S (Table 4.2). Moreover, the presence of the double bond in bis(3,5-dibromosalicyl)fumarate makes it more reactive than its succinyl analog with the same chain length but with a saturated chain.

X-ray crystal-structure analyses of the fumarate and succinate complexes (45) have shown that the cross-linking of Lys β82 groups across the DPG site holds the two β subunits together and prevents them from moving apart as they normally would during the shift to the T state. However, only this region involving the two EF corners is thus constrained. The rest of the tetramer shifts as it normally does in the R-to-T transition. The molecule has nearly its normal oxygen affinity in T and R states in the absence of DPG; the DPG-sensitivity is destroyed because its binding site is occupied. But sickling is impossible because the two acceptor pockets are pulled inward, rather as they are in normal oxyhemoglobin (Figure 4.26). The EF corners no longer have either the correct shape or the correct position to mesh with Val β6 from other molecules and build sickle fibers, even in the deoxygenated state. The specificity for binding to hemoglobin molecules, and the ease with which the bromosalicylate versions can traverse the erythrocyte membrane, make these bifunctional molecules some of the most promising candidates for study, and they are being examined carefully for possible clinical utility.

where R— is: + 2R—OH

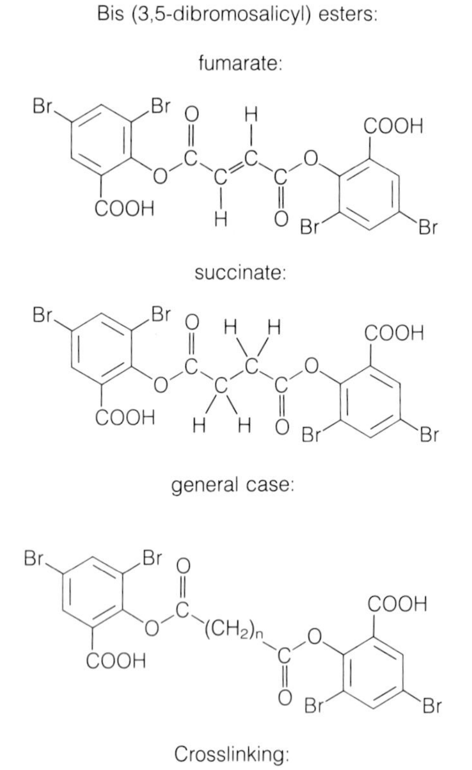

A cure for sickle-cell anemia has not yet been found, but the disease is well understood, to the point where most investigators feel confident that it can be cured. It is truly a molecular disease, and its cure ultimately will come from our understanding of the problem at the molecular level.

One final loose end remains in connection with thalassemias and sickle-cell hemoglobin: Why should heterozygous individuals receive the benefit of protection against malaria, a property that in fact helps both the thalassemic and sickle genes to survive in the human population? The connection between sickle trait and malaria protection was reasonably well established by clinical studies, but that with thalassemic heterozygotes was more tenuous, resting mainly on geographical distribution arguments (Figure 4.1), until laboratory studies were conducted with cultures of the malarial parasite *Plasmodium falciparum* (5). The protozoan parasite spends part of its life cycle multiplying within the red blood cell. The parasite lowers the pH of the host cell slightly, and this makes the cell more prone to sickling. When sickling occurs, the cell membrane becomes more permeable to potassium ions, which leak out into the surroundings. This drop in potassium-ion concentration kills the parasite; if the cells are placed in a high-potassium medium the parasites survive even though the cell sickles. The story with cells from thalassemic heterozygotic carriers is similar in outline. The membrane of a thalassemic cell is more sensitive to damage by oxidation than that of a normal cell, and the hydrogen peroxide generated by the parasite weakens the membrane. It becomes more permeable to potassium ions, and once again the parasite is the agent of its own demise. Hence both sickle trait and thalassemic carrier individuals gain a marginal benefit in malaria resistance because their metabolic disorders confer extra instability on those red blood cells that are infected with parasites, leading to the destruction of at least some of the parasites.

TABLE 4.2 SOLUBILITIES OF NATIVE VERSUS CROSS-LINKED DEOXYHEMOGLOBINS

Derivative	Solubility (g/L)
Native Hb S	163
Succinate (C4 cross-link)	241
Glutarate (C5 cross-link)	198
Adipate (C6 cross-link)	168

Figure 4.34 When two Lys β82 side chains are connected by bis(3,5-dibromosalicyl)-fumarate or succinate (see Figure 4.33) in oxyhemoglobin S, the β subunits are prevented from shifting into their normal deoxyhemoglobin positions upon deoxygenation (see Figure 4.26). Hence the acceptor pocket depicted in Figures 4.23–4.25 cannot reform, and aggregation of molecules into sickled fibers is prevented. This view is a blowup of the F helical portion of a β₁ subunit in Figure 4.18.

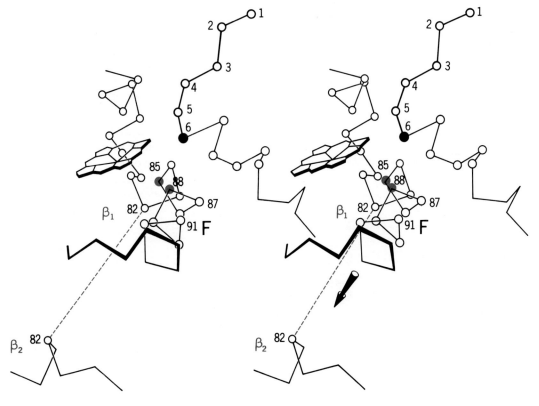

Figure 4.35 Location of all currently known point mutations in α and β human hemoglobin chains. All mutations are shown, both those that produce clinical symptoms and those that were only found during routine electrophoretic screening. Heavy black circles in α_1 and β_2 subunits mark all mutations observed as of 1981. Those human mutant positions that are so essential that they are evolutionarily invariant throughout the long history of the vertebrates are marked by solid color dots, and those additional positions that are invariant if only mammals are considered are given a lighter color tint. (Mutant data from the International Hemoglobin Information Center, Medical College of Georgia, Augusta, Georgia. For information on invariant positions, see Appendix 3.2.)

Although sickle-cell anemia was the first and remains the most studied of molecular disorders caused by point mutations, it is not the only one. Many other abnormal hemoglobins are known with point mutations, or with deletions or insertions of chain. Some have been detected because they give rise to illness or pathological conditions. Changing Glu β121 to Gln (hemoglobin D Los Angeles) or to Lys (hemoglobin O Arab) aggravates the severity of sickling in heterozygous S/D and S/O patients (one hemoglobin S gene and one of hemoglobin D or O) because it strengthens the axial contacts along the sickle fiber (Figure 4.20). Other mutations affect the oxygen-binding properties of the tetramer, or make the molecule unstable and easily denatured. Still others are neutral; they produce no untoward symptoms in their host, and only are discovered during routine electrophoretic screening of blood samples because they change the total charge on the molecule. Many other mutations surely are missed entirely in the human population because they produce no ill effects and we have no easy and routine way of detecting them.

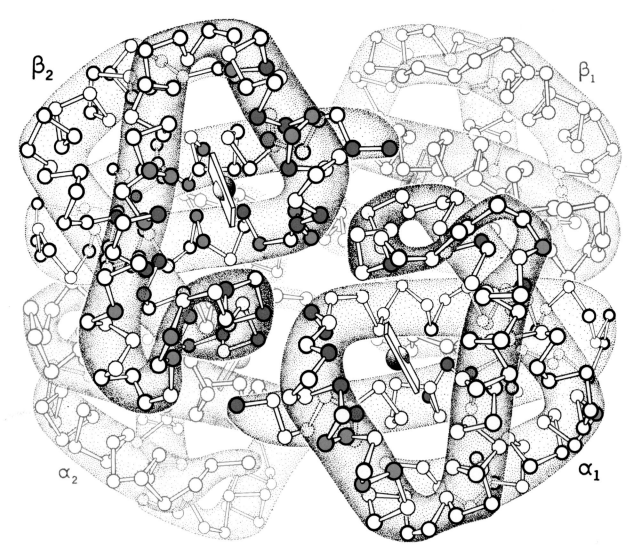

Figure 4.35 shows the locations of all the hemoglobin mutations that have been found as of 1981, whether they show any pathological effect or not. The mutations, plotted as heavy black circles on the closest two subunits only,* are widely scattered over the molecule, indicating that there is no intrinsic tendency for mutations to occur more often at one place in the gene than another. Some idea of the relative importance of these observed mutations to a properly operating hemoglobin molecule can be gained by dividing them into three groups: invariant in all known vertebrate species (dark color dots), invariant in mammals but not so in vertebrates as a whole (light color dots), and evolutionarily variable (uncolored dark rings). Mutations at evolutionarily invariant positions cluster around the heme pockets and intersubunit contacts. As shown by the colored dots in the chapter opening illustration, most of the pathological mutations are also found here. Mutations at variable positions are scattered over the outer surface of the molecule (open circles in Figure 4.35), and these mutations generally have little or no effect on hemoglobin behavior, with the striking exception of the mutation at β6.

Aside from sickle-cell hemoglobin and its relatives, mutant hemoglobins with altered properties generally are of four types:

1. Hemoglobins M, strongly favoring the methemoglobin or oxidized iron state. These usually involve a change in ligation of the heme iron.

2. Hemoglobins with increased oxygen affinity, often because of destabilization of the deoxy or T configuration.

3. Hemoglobins with decreased oxygen affinity, frequently because of damage to the oxy or R configuration.

4. Unstable hemoglobins, usually involving an opening up of the heme pocket, loss of heme, and subsequent precipitation of apohemoglobin in granular deposits (known as Heinz bodies) within the erythrocyte.

These categories are not mutually exclusive; some mutations that damage the heme pockets simultaneously favor oxidation of iron and loss of heme, making the hemoglobin both M and unstable by the foregoing classification. Other mutations that shift the oxygen-binding equilibrium by damaging one state or the other simultaneously make the tetramer easier to denature and therefore unstable. Table 4.3 lists the currently known mutants in these categories, and the map of pathological hemoglobins in Figure 4.36 shows their positions. New mutants are constantly being found. Some of the better known and more studied pathological mutants are named and located in Figure 4.37. Figures 4.38–4.42 illustrate some of the mutants that have been studied by x-ray methods.

1. *Hemoglobins M,* strictly speaking, are those mutants that alter His E7 or His F8 around the heme. The letter is also used for one replacement of the Val E11 that is packed against the heme, blocking access to the iron in the β chain only. Other mutants might logically be classed as hemoglobins M because they favor the Fe(III) state, although they are not customarily designated thus. In the β chain, replacing the distal His E7 by Tyr (M Saskatoon) probably stabilizes ferric iron by bringing a lone electron pair from the tyrosyl oxygen up as a sixth ligand. In the corresponding mutation in the α chain (M Boston), the bond

---

*The chapter opening illustration plots human mutations on all four subunits as a redundant but dramatic gesture.

between His F8 and iron is broken, and the mutant Tyr E7 actually serves as the fifth heme ligand (A6). This is diagrammed in Figure 4.38. Replacing His F8 by Tyr in the α chain (M Iwate) appears from x-ray analysis to cause the heme to become liganded both to Tyr F8 and His E7, but in the β chain (M Hyde Park), ligation is disrupted and 20–30% of the hemes are lost (A12). Replacing Val E11 in the β chain by the negatively charged Glu (M Milwaukee) helps to stabilize the ferric iron (A8), as can be seen in Figure 4.40. (Recall that a ferrous iron in a heme group has a zero net charge, and a ferric iron in a heme has a charge of +1.)

Figure 4.36 Pathological mutations in human hemoglobin. Numbered positions correspond to the colored dots in the chapter-opening illustration on page 116. Black dot: hemoglobin S or sickle mutation. Heavy black ring: hemoglobins M. Dark color: increased oxygen affinity. Light color: decreased oxygen affinity. Jagged perimeter: unstable hemoglobin. Note the similarity between the pattern of pathologies in this figure and the pattern of invariant residues at mutation loci in Figure 4.35. (Data from Table 4.3.)

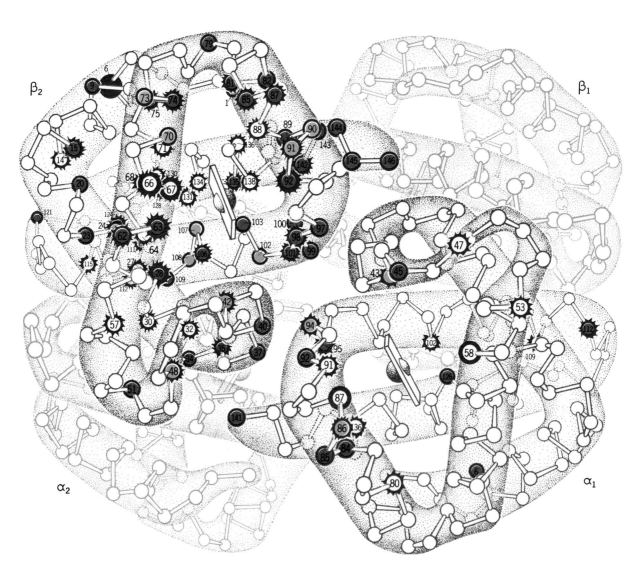

2. Seventy-five of the mutations in Table 4.3 *increase oxygen affinity,* usually by favoring the R state of the tetramer. In many cases the disruption is so severe that the molecule also is unstable. Some mutations increase oxygen affinity by disrupting the network of bonds found at the two chain termini in the T state as shown in Figure 2.24 (Tarrant, Suresnes, and Legnano in the α chain; Olympia, Freiburg, Hirose, Creteil, Andrew-Minneapolis, Bethesda, Rainier, Hiroshima, and others in the β chain). The three α-chain mutations are particularly interesting because they destroy an important Asp H9 to Arg HC3 salt bridge in the deoxy state (Figure 2.24) by eliminating either one side chain or the other. Some mutations increase O_2 affinity because they impair DPG binding by adding a negative charge at the binding site (Shepherds Bush, Ohio), by eliminating a positive charge (Rahere, Helsinki, Little Rock, Syracuse), or by introducing a too-bulky side chain (Abruzzo). Hemoglobin Zurich (Figure 4.41 on page 156) opens the heme pocket to oxygenation by replacing His E7 with the bulkier Arg, which is forced by virtue of its size and its charge to twist out into the solution. Hemoglobin Heathrow distorts the heme pocket by replacing a large Phe at the bottom of the pocket by the smaller Leu. Hemoglobins Chesapeake, J Capetown, Wood, and Malmö favor the T-to-R transition by stabilizing the R state; x-ray studies show deviations from the normal hemoglobin structure in oxy but not in deoxy. But the more common pattern is destabilization of the T state, as we have seen.

Five mutations at βG1 eliminate the βG1(99) to αG4(97) hydrogen bond that is found only in the deoxy state (Figure 2.22), and four others change the chain folding at G2 by removing a Pro (Georgia, Denmark Hill, and Rampa in α, Brigham in β). Hemoglobin Philly eliminates a hydrogen bond by replacing Tyr C1 by Phe, and hemoglobin San Diego introduces a larger nonpolar group into the $\alpha_1\beta_1$ packing-contact surface, both changes being more disruptive in the deoxy configuration. Val βFG5 is important in the T state. It is one means of transmission of information about the heme shift to the FG corner, and its carbonyl group forms a hydrogen bond to Tyr HC2 that is broken during the shift to the R state. Replacing this critical Val by a side chain of the wrong size, either larger (Met) or smaller (Gly, Ala), upsets the T state and hence increases the oxygen affinity of hemoglobin (Köln, Nottingham, Djelfa). In all of the foregoing mutants, the oxygen affinity is increased, and in many of them the molecule is made less stable also.

3. Fewer mutants are known that *decrease oxygen affinity;* Table 4.3 lists 24. Replacing Phe CD1 with a nonaromatic side chain (Torino in α, Hammersmith and Louisville in β) both lowers the oxygen affinity of the molecule and weakens it, probably because the heme must rest against the phenylalanine as it slides and tilts from deoxy to oxy configurations. In Agenogi a salt link between the mutant Lys and the carboxyl terminus traps Tyr HC2 in place and favors the deoxy state. Hemoglobins Kansas and Beth Israel, which eliminate the βG4 to αG1 hydrogen bond of the R state, are the logical inverse of the five mutants mentioned previously that increase oxygen affinity by deleting the βG1 to αG4 bond of the T state. Hemoglobins Yoshizuka, Presbyterian, and Peterborough upset the $\alpha_1\beta_1$ packing contact in ways that are more detrimental in oxy than in deoxy. For the other mutants listed in Table 4.3(IV), it is easier to see why they destabilize the molecule, than why they favor the deoxy state over oxy.

Table 4.3 which begins on page 151 is a seven page list of point mutations that produce abnormal human hemoglobins.

4. The *unstable hemoglobins* in Table 4.3 have many different causes. Many are unstable because an α helix is interrupted and distorted by insertion of proline in the middle (Bibba, Saki, Genova, Perth, Duarte, Bicetre, Mizuho, Atlanta, Santa Ana, Sabine, Southampton, Madrid, Altdorf, Brockton, and Toyoake). Substitution by a too-small amino acid side chain can cause trouble (Torino, Tacoma, Hammersmith, Bucuresti, Sydney, Christchurch, Buenos Aires, Nottingham, Djelfa), as can the insertion of a side chain that is too large (Setif, Riverdale-Bronx, Savannah, Moscva, Zurich, J Calabria, Köln, Peterborough). Introduction of a charged or very polar group inside the molecule or at a subunit contact can be disruptive (Ann Arbor, Moabit, St. Lukes, Manitoba, Suan-Dok, Belfast, Volga, St. Louis, Castilla, Okaloosa, Bristol, Shepherds Bush, Pasadena, Baylor, Boras, Caribbean, Tübingen, Indianapolis, Khartoum, J Guantanamo, Wien, North Shore, Hope). Finally, deletions of single residues or sections of chain are obvious candidates for destabilization of the molecule (Leiden, Niteroi, Tochigi, St. Antoine, Tours, Gun Hill, Leslie).

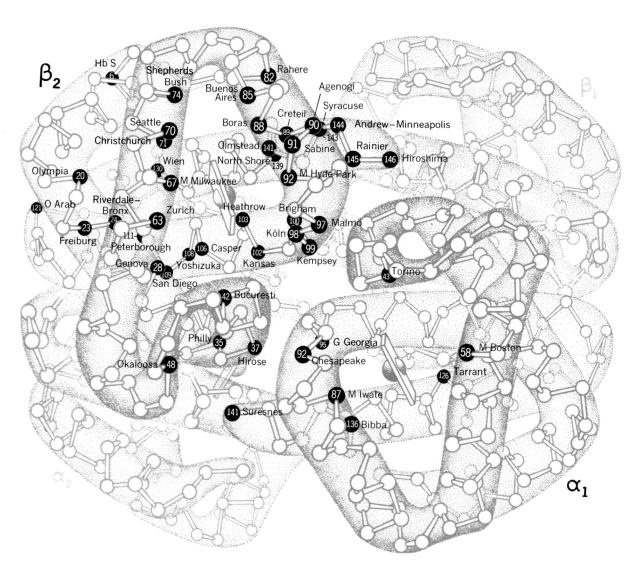

Figure 4.37 Location of some of the most frequently discussed pathological hemoglobin mutants. Note that this and Figure 4.36 reveal that most of the pathological mutations are found on the β chain rather than the α. This probably is so because we possess duplicate α-globin genes, so if one is damaged by mutation the other can produce enough normal chains for survival. Harmful mutations also tend to cluster around the heme pockets and intersubunit contacts, the "active sites" of the hemoglobin molecule.

TABLE 4.3 POINT MUTATIONS THAT PRODUCE ABNORMAL HUMAN HEMOGLOBINS[a,b]

Residue[c]	Change	Name	Consequences and comments
I. SICKLE CELL AND ASSOCIATED FORMS—β CHAIN			
6(A3)	Glu→Val	S	Sickling (XRD).
6(A3)	Glu→Lys	C	Enhances sickling in S/C heterozygote (XRD).
6(A3)	Glu→Ala	G Makassar	
121(GH4)	Glu→Gln	D Los Angeles, D Punjab, D North America, D Portugal, Oak Ridge, D Chicago	Enhances sickling in S/D heterozygote.
121(GH4)	Glu→Lys	O Arab, Egypt	Enhances sickling in S/O heterozygote.
II. HEMOGLOBIN M (FERRIC IRON)			
A. α CHAIN			
58(E7)	His→Tyr	M Boston, M Osaka, Gothenburg, M Kiskunhalas	DEC; heme liganded to Tyr E7, not His F8 (XRD).
● 87(F8)	His→Tyr	M Iwate, M Kankakee, M Oldenburg	FERRI; DEC; heme liganded to both Tyr F8 and E7 (XRD).
B. β CHAIN			
● 28(B10)	Leu→Gln	St. Louis	FERRI; INC; UN; polar substitution tends to open heme pocket (XRD).
63(E7)	His→Tyr	M Saskatoon, M Emory, M Kurume, M Hida, M Radom, M Arhus, M Chicago, Leipzig, Hörlein-Weber, Novi Sad, M Erlangen	FERRI; INC; Tyr ligand stabilizes Fe(III).
● 63(E7)	His→Pro	Bicetre	UN; auto-oxidizing; Pro disrupts center of helix E.
66(E10)	Lys→Glu	I Toulouse	FERRI; UN; replacement of positive charge by negative stabilizes Fe(III).
67(E11)	Val→Glu	M Milwaukee-I	FERRI; DEC; negative charge stabilizes Fe(III) (XRD).
70(E14)	Ala→Asp	Seattle	Charge repels O_2 and stabilizes Fe(III). Side chain opposes heme tilt of T state.
● 92(F8)	His→Tyr	M Hyde Park, M Akita	FERRI; His–heme bond disrupted, 25% heme loss (XRD).

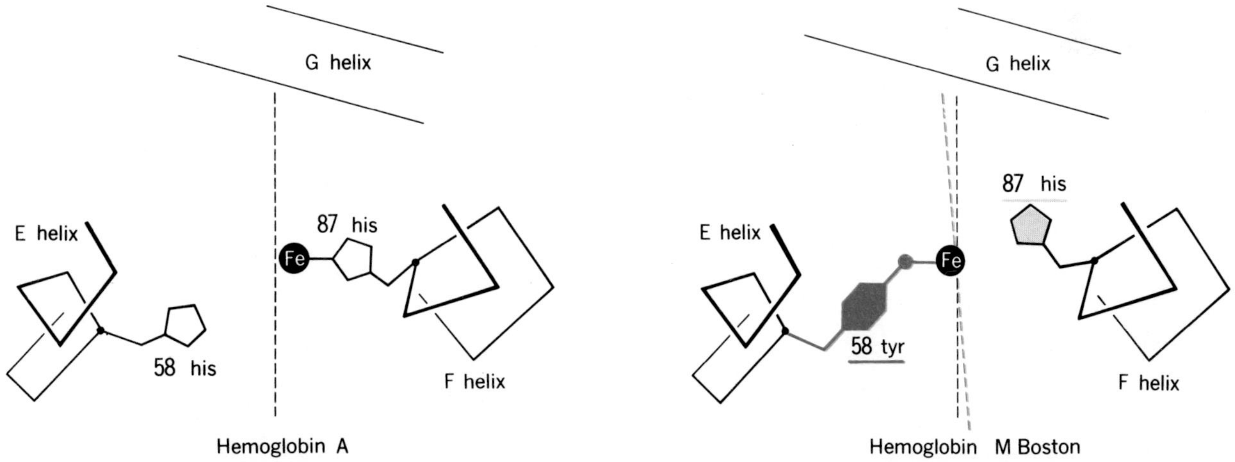

Figure 4.38 Alteration of the heme and surroundings in hemoglobin M Boston, in which His α58(E7) is replaced by Tyr. Normal molecule at the left, mutant at right in colored solid line. The tyrosine becomes the fifth heme ligand in the mutant, the heme moves toward it, and the former heme ligand, His α87(F8), moves away from the heme. With the coupling between heme and F helix broken, the subunits remain in the T configuration, so the oxygen affinity of all subunits is decreased. (From Figure 15 of the Fermi-Perutz *Atlas*.)

● Colored bullets indicate evolutionarily invariant positions (see Figure 3.2).

III. INCREASED O₂ AFFINITY (INC)

A. α CHAIN

6(A4)	Asp→Ala	Sawara	
6(A4)	Asp→Asn	Dunn	
45(CE3)	His→Arg	Fort de France	Salt bridge to heme propionate favors R.
84(F5)	Ser→Arg	Etobicoke	Positive charge on inner side of helix F.
85(F6)	Asp→Asn	G Norfolk	
92(FG4)	Arg→Gln	J Capetown	Slight stabilization of R state (XRD).
92(FG4)	Arg→Leu	Chesapeake	Substitution stabilizes R state (XRD).
● 95(G2)	Pro→Leu	G Georgia	Dissociation ⎫
● 95(G2)	Pro→Ala	Denmark Hill	⎬ Alters chain geometry at subunit contact.
● 95(G2)	Pro→Ser	Rampa	Dissociation ⎭
112(G19)	His→Asp	Hopkins-II	UN
● 126(H9)	Asp→Asn	Tarrant	Eliminates bond to Arg 141 in deoxy.
● 141(HC3)	Arg→His	Suresnes	Eliminates bond to Asn 126 in deoxy (XRD).
● 141(HC3)	Arg→Leu	Legnano	Eliminates bond to Asn 126 in deoxy.

B. β CHAIN

9(A6)	Ser→Cys	Porto Alegre	Polymerization; diminished heme–heme cooperativity.
15(A12)	Trp→Arg	Belfast	UN; bulk replaced by positive charge at contact with helix E.
17–18	(Lys-Val)→O	Lyon	
20(B2)	Val→Met	Olympia	Possibly alters AB bend, disturbing N-terminal bonds in deoxy?
23(B5)	Val→O	Freiburg	Shifts A, B helices, breaks terminal bonds, favors oxy or met.
● 28(B10)	Leu→Gln	St. Louis	FERRI; UN; polar substitution tends to open heme pocket and oppose T state heme tilt. (XRD).
● 28(B10)	Leu→Pro	Genova	UN; substitution alters packing in heme pocket between helices B and E.

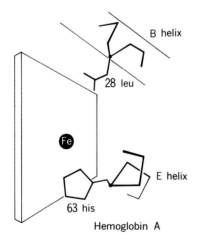

Hemoglobin A

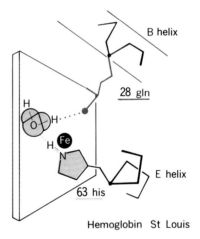

Hemoglobin St Louis

Figure 4.39 Molecular changes in the mutant hemoglobin St. Louis, in which the very polar Gln replaces the hydrophobic Leu at position β28(B10). Normal molecule at left; mutant changes as established by x-ray analysis in color at right. Portions of the B and E helices are at upper and lower right, with the heme plane at left. Position B10 is an interior locus, always hydrophobic in all normal vertebrate globins: Val in rabbit α and Leu in all other chains. Replacement by Gln disrupts the hydrophobic interior and attracts a water molecule into the heme pocket. The water molecule, in turn, bridges to the His 63(E7) side chain and shifts its position. The mutant molecule is thermally unstable and has an increased oxygen affinity. The instability probably arises from introduction of polarity into the molecular interior, and the increased O₂ affinity is thought to arise because the Gln side chain and water molecule interfere with a shift of heme position from that of the R to the T state. (Adapted from Figure 18 of the Fermi-Perutz *Atlas*.)

	Position	Substitution	Name	Description
	34(B16)	Val→Phe	Pitie-Salpetriere	
●	35(C1)	Tyr→Phe	Philly	UN; loss of H-bond favors R state and high O₂ affinity even in deoxy.
●	37(C3)	Trp→Ser	Hirose	Helps free Tyr 145 in deoxy, favoring oxy.
●	40(C6)	Arg→Lys	Athens-Ga, Waco	Disturbs subunit packing in flexible joint.
●	40(C6)	Arg→Ser	Austin	Dissociation; disturbs subunit packing in flexible joint.
	51(D2)	Pro→Arg	Willamette	Positive charge on inner side of helix D.
	62(E6)	Ala→Pro	Duarte	UN; Pro interrupts helix E.
●	63(E7)	His→Tyr	M Saskatoon, etc.	See hemoglobin M.
●	63(E7)	His→Arg	Zürich	UN; Arg swings out, opens O₂ pocket (XRD).
	74(E18)	Gly→Asp	Shepherds Bush	UN; anion repels DPG, favoring oxy (XRD).
	75(E19)	Leu→Arg	Pasadena	UN; introduces charge into hydrophobic corner.
	79(EF3)	Asp→Gly	G-Hsi-Tsou	
	81(EF5)	Leu→Arg	Baylor	UN; introduces charge into hydrophobic corner.
●	82(EF6)	Lys→Thr	Rahere	Eliminates positive charge for DPG binding.
●	82(EF6)	Lys→Met	Helsinki	
	85(F1)	Phe→Ser	Bryn Mawr, Buenos Aires	UN; polar group in heme pocket.
	87(F3)	Thr→O	Tours	UN; shortens chain and disturbs F helix.
●	89(F5)	Ser→Asn	Creteil	Probably disturbs packing of H helix, weakens C-terminal bonds in deoxy (XRD).
	91–95	(Leu-His-Cys-Asp-Lys)→O	Gun Hill	UN; radically shortens F helix near FG corner.
●	92(F8)	His→Gln	St. Etienne, Istanbul	UN; dissociation; His–heme bond disrupted.
●	97(FG4)	His→Gln	Malmö	Slight stabilization of R state.
●	97(FG4)	His→Leu	Wood	
●	98(FG5)	Val→Met	Köln, San Francisco (Pacific), Ube-I	UN
●	98(FG5)	Val→Gly	Nottingham	UN — Substitution alters critical heme contact.
●	98(FG5)	Val→Ala	Djelfa	UN
	99(G1)	Asp→Asn	Kempsey	
	99(G1)	Asp→His	Yakima	(XRD)
	99(G1)	Asp→Ala	Radcliffe	Breaks deoxy intersubunit bonds to αC7 and αG4.
	99(G1)	Asp→Tyr	Ypsilanti	
	99(G1)	Asp→Gly	Hotel-Dieu	
	100(G2)	Pro→Leu	Brigham	Changes chain geometry at subunit contact.
	101(G3)	Glu→Lys	British Columbia	
	101(G3)	Glu→Gly	Alberta	Alters side-chain size in switch region.
	101(G3)	Glu→Asp	Potomac	
●	103(G5)	Phe→Leu	Heathrow	Smaller chain at bottom of heme pocket.
	106(G8)	Leu→Pro	Southampton, Casper	UN; interrupts helix G, alters bottom of heme pocket.
	106(G8)	Leu→Gln	Tübingen	UN; introduces polar group in bottom of heme pocket.
	109(G11)	Val→Met	San Diego	Larger chain disturbs α₁β₁ packing contact, more serious in deoxy (XRD).
	121(GH4)	Glu→Gln	D Los Angeles, D Punjab, D North Carolina, D Portugal, Oak Ridge, D Chicago	
	124(H2)	Pro→Gln	Ty Gard	
	135(H13)	Ala→Pro	Altdorf	UN; interrupts helix H, breaks up C-terminal interactions in T state.
	136(H14)	Gly→Asp	Hope	Asp binds N terminus, decreases DPG affinity.
	142(H20)	Ala→Pro	Toyoake	UN; interrupts helix H, breaks up C-terminal interactions in T state.
	142(H20)	Ala→Asp	Ohio	Anion repels DPG, favoring R state.
	143(H21)	His→Arg	Abruzzo	Bulky side chain at DPG binding site.

143(H21)	His→Gln	Little Rock	Eliminates positive charge for DPG binding.
143(H21)	His→Pro	Syracuse	
144(HC1)	Lys→Asn	Andrew-Minneapolis	Probably disturbs C-terminal bonds in deoxy.
● 145(HC2)	Tyr→His	Bethesda	Upsets C-terminal bonds, favoring R state.
● 145(HC2)	Tyr→Cys	Rainier	Alkali resistant; forms disulfide bridge; (XRD).
● 145(HC2)	Tyr→Asp	Fort Gordon, Osler, Nancy	Upsets C-terminal bonds (XRD).
● 145(HC2)	Tyr→Term	McKees Rocks	Eliminates C-terminal bonds.
● 146(HC3)	His→Asp	Hiroshima	Disrupts T state salt bridge and eliminates Bohr proton source (XRD).
● 146(HC3)	His→Pro	York	Disrupts T state salt bridge and eliminates Bohr proton source.
● 146(HC3)	His→Leu	Cowtown	

IV. DECREASED O₂ AFFINITY (DEC)

A. α CHAIN

● 43(CD1)	Phe→Val	Torino	UN; Phe assists oxy heme tilt; removal favors T state.
58(E7)	His→Tyr	M Boston, etc.	See hemoglobin M.
86(F7)	Leu→Arg	Moabit	UN; introduces charge into invariantly hydrophobic corner of heme pocket.
● 87(F8)	His→Tyr	M-Iwate, etc.	See hemoglobin M.
● 94(G1)	Asp→Asn	Titusville	Dissociation; alters intersubunit bond to αG4 in R state.

B. β CHAIN

1(NA1)	Val→Ac-Ala	Raleigh	Dissociation; deletes positive charge and introduces bulky acetyl group at N terminus.
● 24(B6)	Gly→Asp	Moscva	UN; upsets close contact with Gly E8.
● 42(CD1)	Phe→Ser	Hammersmith, Chiba	UN
● 42(CD1)	Phe→Leu	Louisville, Bucuresti	UN — Phe assists oxy heme tilt; removal favors deoxy.
42–44 or 43–45	(Phe-Glu-Ser)→O or (Glu-Ser-Phe)→O	Niteroi	UN; drastically alters subunit contacts at flexible joint.
48(CD7)	Leu→Arg	Okaloosa	UN; replaces invariant hydrophobic group by positive charges.
67(E11)	Val→Glu	M Milwaukee	See hemoglobin M.
70(E14)	Ala→Asp	Seattle	Charged group at heme contact opens pocket (XRD).

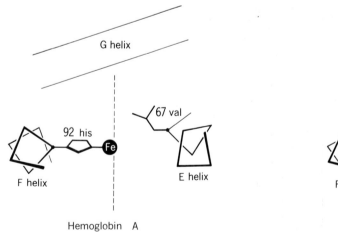
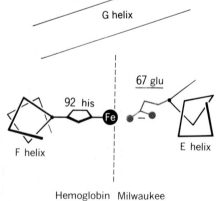

Figure 4.40 In hemoglobin M Milwaukee, Val β67(E11) is replaced by Glu. X-ray analysis shows that the negatively charged Glu side chain forms a bond with the heme iron that stabilizes the Fe(III) state. (From Figure 16 of Fermi and Perutz.)

73(E17)	Asp→Tyr	Vancouver ⎫	Replaces surface negative charge by bulk or
73(E17)	Asp→Val	Mobile ⎭	hydrophobicity.
● 82(EF6)	Lys→Asn→Asp	Providence	
90(F6)	Glu→Lys	Agenogi	Bond to C terminus traps Tyr 145, favoring deoxy.
91(F7)	Leu→Arg	Caribbean	UN; introduces charge into invariantly hydrophobic corner of heme pocket.
102(G4)	Asn→Thr	Kansas ⎫	Dissociation; breaks oxy intersubunit bond to αG1,
102(G4)	Asn→Ser	Beth Israel ⎭	favors deoxy (XRD).
107(G9)	Gly→Arg	Burke	
108(G10)	Asn→Asp	Yoshizuka ⎫	Introduces change in $\alpha_1\beta_1$ contact.
108(G10)	Asn→Lys	Presbyterian ⎭	
111(G13)	Val→Phe	Peterborough	UN; upsets $\alpha_1\beta_1$ contact, worse in oxy.

V. UNSTABLE HEMOGLOBINS (UN)[c]

A. α CHAIN

● 43(CD1)	Phe→Val	Torino	DEC; loss of heme contact. Milder anemia than Hammersmith.
47(CD5)	Asp→His	Hasharon, Sinai, Sealy, L Ferrara	
53(E2)	Ala→Asp	J Rovigo	
80(F1)	Leu→Arg	Ann Arbor	Introduces positive charge into hydrophobic EF corner.
86(F7)	Leu→Arg	Moabit	DEC; introduces charge into invariantly hydrophobic corner of heme pocket.
● 91(FG3)	Leu→Pro	Port Phillip	Rigidifies geometry of chain at FG corner.
● 94(G1)	Asp→Tyr	Setif	Alters subunit contacts at flexible joint.
● 95(G2)	Pro→Arg	St. Lukes	Dissociation; alters chain geometry at subunit contact.
102(G9)	Ser→Arg	Manitoba	Positive charge at bottom of heme pocket.
109(G16)	Leu→Arg	Suan-Dok	Positive charge at contact with helix B.
112(G19)	His→Asp	Hopkins-II	INC
● 136(H19)	Leu→Pro	Bibba	Dissociation; Pro disrupts helix H.

B. β CHAIN

6 or 7	Glu→O	Leiden	
14(A11)	Leu→Pro	Saki	Pro interrupts helix A.
15(A12)	Trp→Arg	Belfast	INC; bulk replaced by positive charge at contact with helix E.
● 24(B6)	Gly→Arg	Riverdale-Bronx ⎫	Upsets close contact with E helix at E8.
● 24(B6)	Gly→Val	Savannah ⎭	
● 24(B6)	Gly→Asp	Moscva	DEC; upsets close contact with E helix at E8.
27(B9)	Ala→Asp	Volga, Drenthe	Negative charge on inside surface of helix.
● 28(B10)	Leu→Gln	St. Louis	FERRI; INC; very polar group in heme pocket (XRD).
● 28(B10)	Leu→Pro	Genova	INC; Pro interrupts helix B, alters contact with helix E.
30(B12)	Arg→Ser	Tacoma	Decreased Bohr and heme–heme; normal O_2 affinity.
32(B14)	Leu→Pro	Perth, Abraham Lincoln	Pro interrupts helix B.
32(B14)	Leu→Arg	Castilla	Positive charge in molecular interior.
● 35(C1)	Tyr→Phe	Philly	INC; loss of $\alpha_1\beta_1$ H bond favors monomers and precipitation (XRD).
● 42(CD1)	Phe→Ser	Hammersmith, Chiba	DEC; loss of heme. Water attracted into pocket.
● 42(CD1)	Phe→Leu	Louisville, Bucuresti	DEC; heme misorientation, but no loss or H_2O. Milder anemia.
42–44 or 43–45	(Phe-Glu-Ser)→O or (Glu-Ser-Phe)→O	Niteroi	DEC; drastically alters subunit contacts at flexible joint.
48(CD7)	Leu→Arg	Okaloosa	DEC; charged group inside subunit.
56→59	(Gly-Asn-Pro-Lys)→O	Tochigi	Drastic shortening of helix E beginning.

57(E1)	Asn→Lys	G Ferrara	
62(E6)	Ala→Pro	Duarte	INC; Pro interrupts helix E.
● 63(E7)	His→Arg	Zürich	INC; larger group swings out, opening pocket. Favors FE(III) and heme loss (XRD).
● 63(E7)	His→Pro	Bicetre	Auto-oxidizing; Pro disrupts center of helix E.
64(E8)	Gly→Asp	J Calabria, J Bari, J Cosenza	
66(E10)	Lys→Glu	I Toulouse	FERRI; replacement of positive charge by negative stabilizes Fe(III).
67(E11)	Val→Asp	Bristol	Charged group at heme contact opens pocket.
67(E11)	Val→Ala	Sydney	Smaller group at heme contact. Water enters, weakening heme pocket (XRD).
68(E12)	Leu→Pro	Mizuho	Pro interrupts helix E.
71(E15)	Phe→Ser	Christchurch	Smaller, polar replacement. Less sensitive than Hammersmith.
74(E18)	Gly→Asp	Shepherds Bush	INC; charged group in EF corner (XRD).
74–75	(Gly-Leu)→O	St. Antoine	Shortens end of helix E.
75(E19)	Leu→Pro	Atlanta	Pro interrupts helix E.
75(E19)	Leu→Arg	Pasadena	INC; introduces charge into hydrophobic corner.
81(EF5)	Leu→Arg	Baylor	INC; introduces charge into hydrophobic corner.
85(F1)	Phe→Ser	Bryn Mawr, Buenos Aires	INC; polar group in heme pocket.
87(F3)	Thr→O	Tours	INC; shortens chain and disturbs F helix.
● 88(F4)	Leu→Arg	Boras	Charged group at heme contact opens pocket.
● 88(F4)	Leu→Pro	Santa Ana ⎫	Helix disruption by Pro.
91(F7)	Leu→Pro	Sabine ⎭	
91(F7)	Leu→Arg	Caribbean	DEC; introduces charge into invariantly hydrophobic corner of heme pocket.
91–95	(Leu-His-Cys-Asp-Lys)→O	Gun Hill	INC; radically shortens F helix near FG corner.
● 92(F8)	His→Gln	St. Etienne, Istanbul	INC; dissociation; ruptures heme attachment. Very polar Gln opens pocket.
● 98(FG5)	Val→Met	Köln, San Francisco (Pacific), Ube-I	INC ⎫
● 98(FG5)	Val→Gly	Nottingham	INC ⎬ Substitution alters critical heme contact.
● 98(FG5)	Val→Ala	Djelfa	INC ⎭

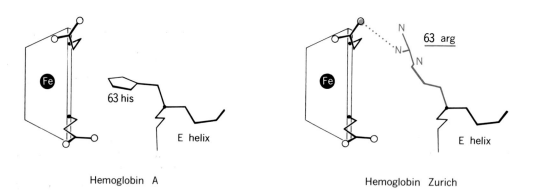

Hemoglobin A   Hemoglobin Zurich

Figure 4.41   In hemoglobin Zürich, His β63(E7) is replaced by Arg. X-ray analysis reveals that the Arg side chain is attracted to the negatively charged propionate chains of the heme on the outside of the molecule, opening up the heme pocket and exposing the iron atom to oxidation to the met state. The increased carbon monoxide affinity of hemoglobin Zürich suggests that in normal hemoglobin A, steric constraints of the side chains around the O_2 binding site favor the O_2 molecule, which binds at an angle to the heme plane, over CO, whose axis lies perpendicular to the heme. Hence the side chains have been tailored by natural selection to discriminate between favorable and unfavorable molecular binding to the heme. (From Figure 19 of Fermi and Perutz.)

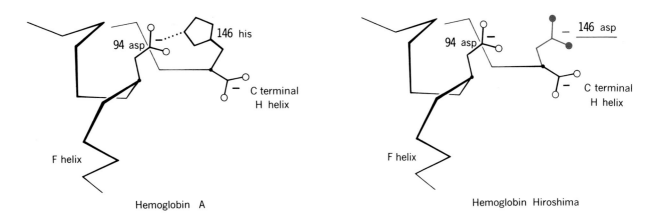

Figure 4.42 In hemoglobin Hiroshima, His β146(HC3) is replaced by Asp. This ruptures a critical salt bridge that stabilizes the T state and provides nearly half of the Bohr protons during the T-to-R conversion. Hence hemoglobin Hiroshima has an increased oxygen affinity and a decreased Bohr effect.

101(G3)	Glu→Gln	Rush	
106(G8)	Leu→Pro	Southampton, Casper	INC; Pro interrupts helix G.
106(G8)	Leu→Gln	Tübingen	INC; introduces polar group in bottom of heme pocket.
111(G13)	Val→Phe	Peterborough	DEC; upsets α₁β₁ contact at β112.
112(G14)	Cys→Arg	Indianapolis	Positive charge in molecular interior.
115(G17)	Ala→Pro	Madrid	Pro interrupts helix G.
124(H2)	Pro→Arg	Khartoum	Positive charge at $\alpha_1\beta_1$ subunit contact.
128(H6)	Ala→Asp	J Guantanamo	Negative charge at $\alpha_1\beta_1$ subunit contact.
130(H8)	Tyr→Asp	Wien	Charged group in subunit interior.
131(H9)	Gln→O	Leslie, Deaconess	Shortens helix H, disturbs C-terminal contacts.
134(H12)	Val→Glu	North Shore	Negative charge at bottom of heme pocket.
135(H13)	Ala→Pro	Altdorf	INC; interrupts helix H, breaks up C-terminal interactions in T state.
138(H16)	Ala→Pro	Brockton	Pro interrupts helix H.
142(H20)	Ala→Pro	Toyoake	INC; interrupts helix H, breaks up C-terminal interactions in T state.

VI. DISSOCIATION[d]

A. α CHAIN

● 94(G1)	Asp→Asn	Titusville	DEC; alters FG corner subunit contact.
● 95(G2)	Pro→Leu	G Georgia	INC ⎫ Alters chain geometry at subunit contact.
● 95(G2)	Pro→Ser	Rampa	INC ⎭
● 95(G2)	Pro→Arg	St. Lukes	UN; alters chain geometry at subunit contact.
● 136(H19)	Leu→Pro	Bibba	UN; helix disruption by Pro.

B. β CHAIN

1(NA1)	Val→Ac-Ala	Raleigh	DEC; deletes positive charge and introduces bulky acetyl group at N terminus.
● 40(C6)	Arg→Ser	Austin	INC; disturbs subunit packing in flexible joint.
● 92(F8)	His→Gln	St. Etienne, Istanbul	INC; UN; His–heme bond disrupted.
102(G4)	Asn→Thr	Kansas	DEC; breaks oxy intersubunit bond, favors deoxy (XRD).

[a]Excerpted from the International Hemoglobin Information Center Tabulation of February 1981 (Comprehensive Sickle Cell Center, Augusta, Georgia 30912).
[b]INC = increased O_2 affinity; DEC = decreased O_2 affinity; UN = unstable hemoglobin; FERRI = Fe(III) heme favored; XRD = x-ray diffraction analysis available. A good discussion of x-ray analyses of abnormal human hemoglobin is to be found in the Fermi and Perutz *Hemoglobin Atlas*.
[c]These lead to globin precipitation, or Heinz bodies.
[d]All listed have been included in earlier categories.

Whether a mutation at a given site will change the behavior of the hemoglobin depends both on the site and the particular substitution. Replacement of Phe at CD1 by Val (Torino) or Leu (Louisville) is harmful because it removes an important heme-packing contact, leading to an unstable hemoglobin and mild anemia in the host. But replacement by Ser (Hammersmith) is still more serious because the polar hydroxyl group of serine attracts a water molecule into the heme pocket and facilitates denaturation of the molecule. Patients with hemoglobin Hammersmith are seriously anemic. In contrast, replacing Phe by Tyr at C7 in hemoglobin Mequon produces no change in molecular properties; at that position Phe and Tyr are functional synonyms. They are not synonymous if the hydrogen bond of Tyr is important, as hemoglobin Philly at C1 demonstrates. The Ser-for-Phe substitution that is so serious at CD1 in hemoglobin Hammersmith is much less so at E15 in Christchurch, because that site is a less sensitive part of the molecule. In the language of molecular genetics, a mutation changing Phe to Tyr at CD1 has a selection coefficient of nearly zero, mutations changing Phe to Val or Leu have small negative selection coefficients, and a Phe-to-Ser mutation has a large negative selection coefficient because it is so harmful. But the same Phe-to-Ser mutation at E15 has only a slightly negative coefficient.

Sickling is produced by replacing Glu by the nonpolar Val at β6(A3), and is aggravated by the presence of Lys at the same position in the other β gene of heterozygotes (hemoglobin C). But replacing this same Glu by Ala in G Makassar does not create enough of an oily patch to shift the sickling equilibrium; presumably Ala fits less well into the EF acceptor pocket than Val. Outright deletion of position A3 in hemoglobin Leiden also prevents sickling; the shortening of the A helix by one residue and the moving of Pro β5 probably causes a mismatch between the A helix and the EF pocket. The destabilizing effects of replacement of Gly by Asp at E18 in Shepherds Bush must arise from charge rather than size, since insertion of the similarly shaped Val in Bushwick is symptomless.

By now it may seem surprising from Table 4.3 or Figure 4.36 that almost all of the pathological mutations involve the β subunit, whereas Figure 4.35 indicates a much more uniform distribution of all mutations. This probably arises because humans have two α genes but only one β. Even if one of the α genes receives a lethal mutation and the individual is homozygous for that gene, the other α gene on chromosome 16 is there to manufacture normal chains. Although mutations probably occur just as frequently at α genes as at β genes, they are less likely to be pathological. If, as Figure 3.7 suggests, the δ gene is a "spoiled" β gene—spoiled because of too-early shutdown or instability of its messenger—then this inadequacy of the δ gene has exposed us to a host of molecular diseases of the β chain, which we would have escaped had we retained a second functional β gene.

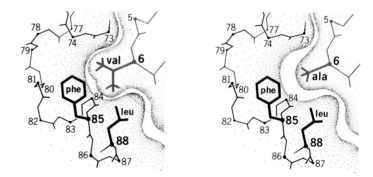

Figure 4.43 In sickled hemoglobin the acceptor pocket for the mutant β6 Val is formed by both Phe 85 and Leu 88. If the β6 donor is Ala rather than Val then two methyl groups are lost, and the contact with the crucial pair 85 and 88 is inadequate.

All of the physiologically functional tetrameric hemoglobins are combinations of two chains from the α family (α or ζ), and two from the β family (β, γ, δ, or ϵ). The most striking structural difference between these two families is the deletion of the D helix and consequent shortening of the CD corner in the α family. Patients with α-thalassemia produce too few α chains, and the excess β-family chains can form homotetramers such as β_4 (hemoglobin H) or γ_4 (hemoglobin Bart's). These homotetramers are useless for oxygen transport. They have a hyperbolic, myoglobin-like oxygen binding curve with no heme–heme cooperativity, and exhibit high oxygen affinity at all physiological oxygen pressures, both at the lungs and at the tissues (48–50). The Bohr effect, or pH dependence on oxygen affinity, is also eliminated. Functionally, hemoglobins H and Bart's behave like four isolated subunits that just happen to be gathered together into one molecular unit. They bind oxygen normally at the lungs, but then cannot release it at the tissues in the way that normal hemoglobin can.

There is good evidence that the β_4 tetramers do not undergo a subunit rearrangement like the T-to-R conversion when they are oxygenated and deoxygenated, and also that their subunits are arranged in hemoglobin H like those of the normal R state rather than the T. Perutz and Mazzarella showed in 1963 that crystals of methemoglobin* H could be reduced in ferrous citrate solution without crystal damage, whereas reduction of methemoglobin A crystals or oxidation of deoxyhemoglobin A crystals always caused them to shatter (51). Hence there cannot be a subunit transition of anything like the magnitude found in normal hemoglobin A. Flash photolysis experiments with carbonmonoxyhemoglobin H also show that only a single species is present to recombine with CO, rather than two as with hemoglobin A.

The crystal symmetry and cell dimensions of hemoglobin H are closer to those of deoxyhemoglobin A than methemoglobin A or carbonmonoxyhemoglobin A, suggesting at first glance that the common structure possessed by the β_4 molecule in both oxygenation states might resemble what now would be termed a normal T state. DPG binds tightly to hemoglobin H, supporting this picture, although it binds equally well to the oxy and deoxy states and has no effect on oxygen binding (49). Most evidence, however, favors an R-like subunit arrangement for the β_4 molecule: the high oxygen affinity itself, the rapid kinetics of oxygen binding and loss, and the reactivity of the sulfhydryl group of Cys β93 in both oxy and deoxy states (48–50). (Cys β93 is protected and unreactive in the T conformation of deoxyhemoglobin A.) Hydrogen–tritium exchange behavior is identical in oxy and deoxyhemoglobin H, and resembles that of oxy rather than deoxyhemoglobin A. The x-ray structure analysis of carbonmonoxyhemoglobin H has revealed that the distances between heme iron atoms are more like those in normal oxy than deoxy (52). Even more significantly, the side chain from FG4 sits between C3 and C6 on a neighboring subunit, like the R state of normal hemoglobin, rather than between C6 and CD2 as in the T state (53). (See Figures 2.20 and 2.21.) Hence, in terms of FG corner/C helix packing, hemoglobin H is in an oxy-like configuration. The similarity of cell dimensions between hemoglobin H and deoxyhemoglobin A was a false trail; the molecular twofold axes are oriented 90° differently in the two structures.

---

*The distinction between oxyhemoglobin and methemoglobin was not always made in the literature at that time, but the context suggests that "oxyhemoglobin" probably was methemoglobin.

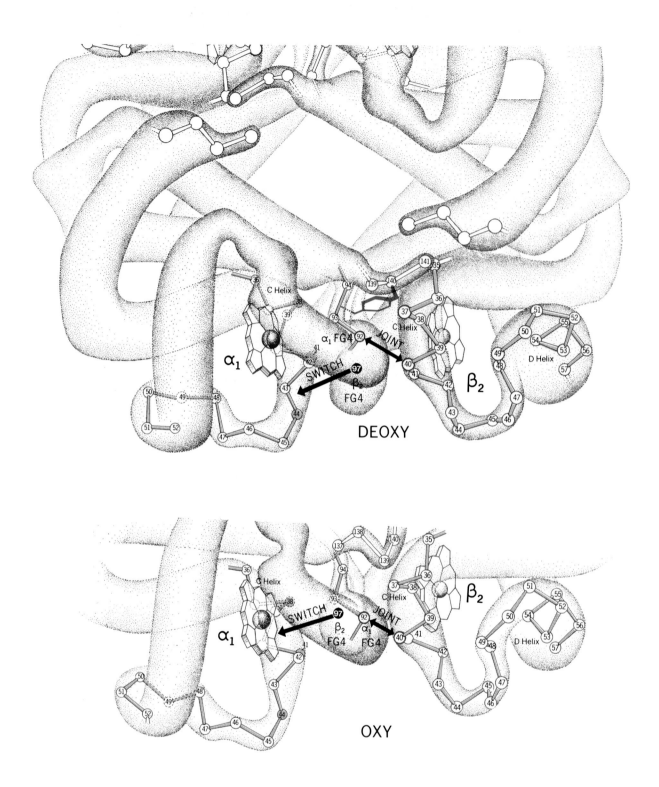

Figure 4.44 Hemoglobin molecule viewed down the twofold axis with α chains on top. Contacts in the flexible joint and switch regions (heavy black arrows) are more alike in the lower drawing of oxyhemoglobin than they are in deoxyhemoglobin above (see text opposite). The βC helix is held firmly against the αFG corner by the pressure of the βD helix at the flexible joint, where the large size of residues Arg α92(FG4) and Arg β40(C6) prevents them from slipping past one another as the analogous chains in the switch region can. Hence the flexible joint is constrained to act as a hinge, rather than a sliding switch.

Other homotetramers from the β family are known, such as γ$_4$ and δ$_4$, but the α chains cannot form tetramers. What is it that forbids α$_4$ tetramers, and why must two of the four chains seemingly be α in order for a tetramer to show heme–heme cooperativity and a Bohr effect? The D helix is suspect at once because it is present in β chains but absent in α. Unfortunately for this most simpleminded interpretation, the D helices of β subunits sit on the surface of the molecule, about as isolated from other subunits as they could be (Figure 4.44). Their real importance probably lies in their effect in positioning the adjacent C helices. The presence of a D helix in the β subunit pushes the C helix of that subunit close to the FG corner of an adjacent α subunit in the flexible-joint region (Figure 4.44). Elimination of the D helix in the α subunit shortens the B-to-E region of chain, and allows a looser packing of the C helix from the α subunit against the FG corner of a neighboring β subunit in the switch region (Figures 2.20 and 2.21).

In normal hemoglobin A, the flexible-joint and switch regions are more alike in oxy than in deoxyhemoglobin, in the sense that the side chain of FG4 sits between side chains of C3 and C6, rather than C6 and CD2. (Compare Figures 2.20 and 2.21 with the adjoining 4.44, and Figures 12 and 13 of reference 54.) Arg α92(FG4) is packed against Arg α40(C6) in the flexible joint, but does not slip past it from one side to the other during the T-to-R transition. In contrast, at the other end of the molecule, the smaller His β97(FG4) slips easily to the other side of the smaller Thr α41(C6) in the switch region with the change in subunit arrangement. Hence the two ends of the hemoglobin A molecules are more nearly alike in the R state than in the T state. In retrospect, therefore, it is only natural that hemoglobin H, in which the two ends of the tetrameric molecule are truly identical, should be found in an R-like conformation. Special pleading would have been required to explain why a tetramer of four identical β chains should exhibit a flexible-joint-like region at one end, and a quite different deoxy-switch-like region at the other.

It is a reasonable assumption that the ancestral globin subunit was more β-like, with subsequent deletion of the D helix in the α family, since myoglobins and monomeric globins all possess a D helix. An ancestral β$_4$ tetramer, like hemoglobin H today, would bring four subunits together and lower the osmotic pressure of the medium, but would show no more cooperative or Bohr effects than would the separated subunits. Two evolutionary adaptations probably were necessary for the development of a tetramer capable of subunit transitions: loosening of the tight packing between C helix and FG corner in the switch region by deletion of the D helices in two of the four chains, and substitution of smaller residues for the two arginines at FG4 (βFG4 is histidine) and C6 (αC6 is threonine) where the side chains would have to move past one another.

The observed hemoglobin subunit motion follows naturally if one assumes only that FG4 is small enough to slip past C6 in the switch region, but too large to do so in the flexible joint. Figure 4.45 is a drastically simplified version of Figure 2.19, with the tetramer viewed down the α$_1$β$_1$ pseudo-twofold axis. Only the C helices and FG4 residues are shown, although these appear in their correct relative positions. Colored lines and ovals represent the α$_2$ and β$_2$ subunits that are below the plane of the page, and black lines and ovals represent the α$_1$ and β$_1$ subunits closer to the viewer. Figure 4.45 shows the oxy structure, and black arrows indicate the motions of α$_1$β$_1$ that occur during the R-to-T transition. The axis of subunit rotation is such that in the switch region the FG4 side chain moves *along* the axis of its opposed C helix, whereas in the joint region it merely moves from one side of the C helix to the other. This constraint in the joint regions and

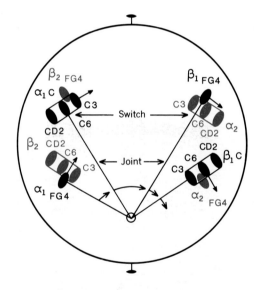

Figure 4.45 Relative positions of C helices and FG corners in oxy- and deoxyhemoglobin. Residues in the α$_2$ and β$_2$ subunits to the rear of the molecule as viewed here are in color, and those in the α$_1$ and β$_1$ subunits closer to the viewer are in black. This is the oxy configuration. Black arrows indicate the motion of the α$_1$β$_1$ dimer in going to the deoxy state. In the switch region at the top of the diagram, residues FG4 and C6 slip past one another, but in the flexible joint beneath it, they merely slide against one another in place. (Compare Figure 2.19.)

looseness in the switch essentially *require* the axis of subunit rotation to pass through the α subunits in the way that is actually observed. In β_4 hemoglobin H, the α D helix pushes its C helix against the β FG corner, freezing the switch and preventing subunit motion. In contrast, when all four D helices are missing, as in an α_4 tetramer, there evidently is too little constraint to keep the subunits from falling apart. One other evolutionary change may have assisted in the development of the R-to-T transition: residue CD2 is invariably Asp in myoglobins, and usually Asp or Glu in β chains. In α chains it usually is Pro, and this uncharged group may encourage the β helix to slide out toward it in the deoxy configuration. (See Figure 2.21.)

The Port Jackson shark seems at first glance to represent an anomaly in this simple story. As the sequence comparisons in Table 3.1 show, the D helix is missing from both the α and the β chains of shark hemoglobin. Furthermore, the differences between a shark α or β chain and the corresponding members of the same α or β family among higher vertebrates are nearly as large as the differences between α and β families themselves (Table 3.3). Shark α differs from all other α by an average of 91(5) residues (mean of 91 and standard deviation of 5) and shark β differs from other β by 95(3). Shark β differs from all α by 97(3), and shark β from all α by 105(3). The divergence of shark from bony fish and all higher vertebrates must have occurred very soon after the separation of α and β genes. Table 3.3 does provide evidence, however, that not all of the differences in shark are simply the accumulation of random changes: shark α chain is more different from β chains than are the α chains of higher vertebrates, although they all should be equally distant from β. Similarly, shark β chain is more different from all α than other β chains are. Evidently there is a real sense in which the shark chains have gone their separate ways from those of higher vertebrates, accumulating more changes than simple neutral mutation theory would predict. One of these special developments seems to have been the elimination of the D helix in the β chain as well as in the α, and it would be extremely interesting to look at the structure of the Port Jackson shark hemoglobin and see what keeps its tetramer together when α_4 tetramers of higher vertebrates are unstable and fall apart.

In summary, the evolution of the functional hemoglobin $\alpha_2\beta_2$ tetramer might be considered to have involved the following three steps:

1. Accumulation of less polar side chains in the region that would ultimately correspond to $\alpha_1\beta_2$ sliding contacts in the R state of the tetramer, leading to a molecule (as in modern lamprey) that dimerizes in the oxy state and dissociates when O_2 is lost.

2. Accumulation of less polar side chains in what ultimately would be the $\alpha_1\beta_1$ packing-contact zones, favoring a β_4 homotetramer frozen in an R-like configuration, with high oxygen affinity but no heme–heme cooperativity, Bohr effect, or sensitivity to effectors such as DPG.

3. Deletion of D helices in two of the four chains (i.e., development of the α gene), and adjustment of size and polarity of residues in the switch region to permit a two-state subunit transition, leading ultimately to heme–heme cooperativity, pH sensitivity, and allosteric control of oxygen binding.

The hemoglobin molecule, in this picture, is the result of as much as a billion years of selective tuning, to produce finally an oxygen carrier with all of the useful properties that we know today.

GENERAL REFERENCES

1. Lehmann, H., and Huntsman, R. G., 1974. *Man's Haemoglobins* (2nd ed.), North-Holland Publishing Company, Amsterdam.
2. Maniatis, T., Fritsch, E. F., Lauer, J., and Lawn, R. M., 1980. *Ann. Rev. Genetics* 14:145–178.
3. Bank, A., Mears, J. G., and Ramirez, F., 1980. *Science* 207:486–493.
4. Kolata, G. B., 1980. *Science* 210:300–302.
5. Friedman, M. J., and Trager, W., 1981. *Scientific American* (Mar.), 154–164.
6. Arnone, A., and Briley, P. D., 1978. In W. S. Caughey (Ed.), *Biochemical and Clinical Aspects of Hemoglobin Abnormalities,* Academic Press, New York, pp. 93–107.
7. Pauling, L., Itano, H. A., Singer, S. J., and Wells, I. C., 1949. *Science* 110:543–548.
8. Ingram, V. M., 1956. *Nature* 178:792–794.
9. Bookchin, R. M., and Nagel, R. L., 1974. *Seminars in Hematology* 11:577–595.
10. Dean, J., and Schechter, A. N., 1978. *New Eng. J. Med.* 299:752–763, 804–811, and 863–870.
11. Noguchi, C. T., and Schechter, A. N., 1981. *Blood,* 58:1057–1068.
12. Murayama, M., 1966. *Science* 153:145–149.
13. Murayama, M., 1966. *J. Cell. Physiol.* 67 (Supplement 1):21–31.
14. Wellems, T. E., and Josephs, R., 1979. *J. Mol. Biol.* 135:651–674.
15. Finch, J. T., Perutz, M. F., Bertles, J. F., and Dobler, J., 1973. *Proc. Natl. Acad. Sci. USA* 70:718–722.
16. Josephs, R., Jarosch, H. S., and Edelstein, S. J., 1976. *J. Mol. Biol.* 102:409–426.
17. Dykes, G., Crepeau, R. H., and Edelstein, S. J., 1978. *Nature* 272:506–510.
18. Crepeau, R. H., Dykes, G., Garrell, R., and Edelstein, S. J., 1978. *Nature* 274:616–617.
19. Dykes, G. W., Crepeau, R. H., and Edelstein, S. J., 1979. *J. Mol. Biol.* 130:451–472.
20. Garrell, R. L., Crepeau, R. H., and Edelstein, S. J., 1979. *Proc. Natl. Acad. Sci. USA* 76:1140–1144.
21. Edelstein, S. J., 1980. *Biophys. J.* 32:347–360.
22. Wellems, T. E., and Josephs, R., 1980. *J. Mol. Biol.* 137:443–450.
23. Wellems, T. E., Vassar, R. J., and Josephs, R., 1981. *J. Mol. Biol.* 153:1011–1026.
24. Josephs, R., Vassar, R. J., Rezenka, A., and Sigler, P., 1981. *Rheological Aspects of Sickle Cell Disease*, Airlie House Symposium, Airlie, Va.
25. Vassar, R. J., Potel, M. J., and Josephs, R., 1982. *J. Mol. Biol.,* 157:395–412.

26. Magdoff-Fairchild, B., and Chiu, C. C., 1979. *Proc. Natl. Acad. Sci. USA* 76:223–226.

27. Pumphrey, J. G., and Steinhardt, J., 1976. *Biochem. Biophys. Res. Commun.* 69:99–105.

28. Pumphrey, J. G., and Steinhardt, J., 1977. *J. Mol. Biol.* 112:359–375.

29. Benesch, R. E., Kwong, S., Benesch, R., and Edalji, R., 1977. *Nature* 269:772–775.

30. Nagel, R. L., and Bookchin, R. M., 1978. In W. S. Caughey (Ed.), *Biochemical and Clinical Aspects of Hemoglobin Abnormalities,* Academic Press, New York, pp. 195–204.

31. Nagel, R. L., Johnson, J., Bookchin, R. M., Garel, M. C., Rosa, J., Schiliro, G., Wajcman, H., Labie, D., Moo-Penn, W., and Castro, O., 1980. *Nature* 283:832–834.

32. Edelstein, S. J., 1981. *J. Mol. Biol.* 150:557–575.

33. Geis, I., Walder, J., Arnone, A., and Dekleva, K., in preparation.

34. Hofrichter, J., Ross, P. D., and Eaton, W. A., 1974. *Proc. Natl. Acad. Sci. USA* 71:4864–4868.

35. Eaton, W. A., Hofrichter, J., and Ross, P. D., 1976. *Blood* 47:621–627.

36. Hofrichter, J., Ross, P. D., and Eaton, W. A., 1976. *Proc. Natl. Acad. Sci. USA* 73:3035–3039.

37. Sunshine, H. R., Hofrichter, J., and Eaton, W. A., 1978. *Nature* 275:238–240.

38. Cooperative Urea Trials Group, 1974. *J. Am. Med. Assn.* 228:1125–1128.

39. Schechter, A. N., and Noguchi, C. T., 1979. *Development of Therapeutic Agents for Sickle-Cell Disease,* INSERM Symposium No. 9, J. Rosa, Y. Beuzard, and J. Hercules (Eds.), Elsevier/North-Holland Biomedical Press, Amsterdam, pp. 129–138.

40. Schechter, A. N., 1980. *Hemoglobin* 4:335–345.

41. Acharya, A. S., and Manning, J. M., 1980. *J. Biol. Chem.* 255:1406–1412.

42. Packer, L., Bymun, E. N., Tinberg, H. M., and Ogunmala, G. B., 1976. *Arch. Biochem. Biophys.* 177:323–329.

43. Klotz, I. M., and Tam, J. W. O., 1973. *Proc. Natl. Acad. Sci. USA* 70:1313–1315.

44. Klotz, I. M., Haney, D. N., and King, L. C., 1981. *Science* 213:724–731.

45. Walder, J. A., Walder, R. Y., and Arnone, A., 1980. *J. Mol. Biol.* 141:195–216.

46. Chatterjee, R., Walder, R. Y., Arnone, A., and Walder, J. A., 1982. *Biochemistry,* in press.

47. Walder, J. A., in preparation.

48. Benesch, R., and Benesch, R. E., 1964. *Nature* 202:773–775.

49. Benesch, R., Benesch, R. E., and Enoki, Y., 1968. *Proc. Natl. Acad. Sci. USA* 61:1102–1106.

50. Benesch, R., and Benesch, R. E., 1974. *Science* 185:905–908.

51. Perutz, M. F., and Mazzarella, L., 1963. *Nature* 199:639.

52. Arnone, A., and Briley, P. D., 1978. In W. S. Caughey (Ed.), *Biochemical and Clinical Aspects of Hemoglobin Abnormalities,* Academic Press, New York.

53. Arnone, A., Briley, P. D., and Rogers, P. H., 1982. In C. Ho (Ed.), *Interaction Between Iron and Proteins in Oxygen and Electron Transport,* Elsevier/North-Holland, New York.

54. Baldwin, J., and Chothia, C., 1979. *J. Mol. Biol.* 129:175–220.

APPENDIX 4.1 MUTANT HEMOGLOBIN STRUCTURE ANALYSES

For explanation, see Appendix 2.1.

Date	Name	Position	Amino acid change	Analysis	References
1975	Hemoglobin S	β6(A3)	E→V	3.0 Mol.	A1, A2
1979	Hemoglobin C	β6(A3)	E→K	?	A3
1976	St. Louis	β28(B10)	L→Q	3.5 ΔF, $\phi_{\text{deoxy A}}$	A4
1977	Tacoma	β30(B12)	R→S	3.5 ΔF, $\phi_{\text{deoxy A}}$	A5
1973	M Boston	α58(E7)	H→Y	3.5 ΔF, $\phi_{\text{deoxy A}}$	A6
1978	Zürich, CO	β63(E7)	H→R	2.8 ΔF, $\phi_{\text{CO HbA}}$	A7
1978	Sydney, CO	β67(E11)	V→A	2.7 ΔF, $\phi_{\text{CO HbA}}$	A7
1972	M Milwaukee	β67(E11)	V→E	3.5 ΔF, $\phi_{\text{deoxy A}}$	A8
1973	Seattle	β70(E14)	A→D	3.5 ΔF, $\phi_{\text{deoxy A}}$	A9
	Shepherds Bush	β74(E18)	G→D	3.5 ΔF, $\phi_{\text{deoxy A}}$	A10
1981	Creteil	β89(F5)	S→N	3.5 ΔF, $\phi_{\text{deoxy A}}$	A11
1971	M Iwate	α87(F8)	H→Y	5.5 MIR	A12
1971	M Hyde Park	β92(F8)	H→Y	3.5 ΔF, $\phi_{\text{deoxy A}}$	A12
1971	Chesapeake	α92(FG4)	R→L	5.5 ΔF, $\phi_{\text{deoxy A}}$	A13
1971	Capetown	α92(FG4)	R→Q	5.5 ΔF, $\phi_{\text{deoxy A}}$	A13
1973	Yakima	β99(G1)	D→H	3.5 ΔF, $\phi_{\text{deoxy A}}$	A14
1971	Kansas	β102(G4)	N→T	3.4 ΔF, $\phi_{\text{deoxy A}}$	A15, A16
1975	Kansas, CO	β102(G4)	N→T	3.4 ΔF, $\phi_{\text{deoxy A}}$	A16
1971	Richmond	β102(G4)	N→L	4.0 ΔF, $\phi_{\text{deoxy A}}$	A15
1974	San Diego	β109(G11)	V→M	3.5 ΔF, $\phi_{\text{deoxy A}}$	A17
	Hope	β136(H14)	G→D	3.5 ΔF, $\phi_{\text{deoxy A}}$	A18
1971	Rainier	β145(HC2)	Y→C	3.5 ΔF, $\phi_{\text{deoxy A}}$	A19
1976	Nancy	β145(HC2)	Y→D	3.5 ΔF, $\phi_{\text{deoxy A}}$	A20
1980	Suresnes	α141(HC3)	R→H	3.5 ΔF, $\phi_{\text{deoxy A}}$	A21
1971	Hiroshima	β146(HC3)	H→D	3.5 ΔF, $\phi_{\text{deoxy A}}$	A22
1976	Cochin-Port Royal	β146(HC3)	H→R	3.5 ΔF, $\phi_{\text{deoxy A}}$	A20

APPENDIX 4.1 REFERENCES

A1. Wishner, B. C., Ward, K. B., Lattman, E. E., and Love, W. E., 1975. *J. Mol. Biol.* 98:179–194.

A2. Wishner, B. C., Hanson, J. C., Ringle, W. M., and Love, W. E., 1976. *Proceedings of the Symposium on Molecular Cellular Aspects of Sickle Cell Disease,* DHEW Publication 76-1007, National Institutes of Health, Bethesda, Md., pp. 1–31.

A3. Love, W. *et al.,* in preparation.

A4. Anderson, N. L., 1976. *J. Clin. Invest.* 58:1107–1109.

A5. Tucker, P. W., and Perutz, M. F., 1977. *J. Mol. Biol.* 114:415–420.

A6. Pulsinelli, P. D., Perutz, M. F., and Nagel, R. L., 1973. *Proc. Natl. Acad. Sci. USA* 70:3870–3874.

A7. Tucker, P. W., Phillips, S. E. V., Perutz, M. F., Houtchens, R., and Caughey, W. S., 1978. *Proc. Natl. Acad. Sci. USA* 75:1076–1080.

A8. Perutz, M. F., Pulsinelli, P. D., and Ranney, H., 1972. *Nature New Biol.* 237:259–264.

A9. Anderson, N. L., Perutz, M. F., and Stamatoyannopoulos, G., 1973. *Nature New Biol.* 243:274–275.

A10. Battison, D., Dintzis, H. M., and Perutz, M. F., in preparation.

A11. Arnone, A., Thillet, J., and Rosa, J., 1981. *J. Biol. Chem.,* in press.

A12. Greer, J., 1971. *J. Mol. Biol.* 59:107–126.

A13. Greer, J., 1971. *J. Mol. Biol.* 62:241–249.

A14. Pulsinelli, P. D., 1973. *J. Mol. Biol.* 74:57–66.

A15. Greer, J., 1971. *J. Mol. Biol.* 59:99–105.

A16. Anderson, N. L., 1975. *J. Mol. Biol.* 94:33–49.

A17. Anderson, N. L., 1974. *J. Clin. Invest.* 53:329–333.

A18. Battison, D., Dintzis, H. M., and Perutz, M. F., in preparation.

A19. Greer, J., and Perutz, M. F., 1971. *Nature New Biol.* 230:261–264.

A20. Arnone, A., Gacon, G., and Wajcman, H., 1976. *J. Biol. Chem.* 251:5875–5880.

A21. Poyart, C., Bursaux, E., Arnone, A., Bonaventura, J., and Bonaventura, C., 1980. *J. Biol. Chem.* 255:9465–9473.

A22. Perutz, M. F., Pulsinelli, P. D., Ten Eyck, L., Kilmartin, J. V., Shibata, S., Iuchi, I., Miyaji, T., and Hamilton, H. B., 1971. *Nature New Biol.* 232:147–149.

APPENDIX 4.2 INTERSUBUNIT CONTACTS IN DEOXYHEMOGLOBIN S CRYSTALS[a]

[a]*Numbers in the body of this table are the number of pairwise approaches of 5 Å or less between atoms of side chains on different subunits. Numbers to left and right of slashes in A and B are for corresponding but nonidentical contacts on opposite strands. (From E. Padlan and W. Love, private communication, 1981.) This table provided the data for Figures 4.20 and 4.21b.*

A. LATERAL CONTACTS

			1 or 2 β1															Heme
			E helix					EF corner					F helix					
			Lys 66	Gly 69	Ala 70	Phe 71	Asp 73	His 77	Asp 79	Asa 80	Gly 83	Thr 84	Phe 85	Thr 87	Leu 88	Glu 90	Leu 91	
2 or 1 α2	B helix	Leu 34						—/2										
	CD corner	Ser 49							1/6									
		His 50							—/3	15/—								
2 or 1 β2	A helix	Thr 4				7/4												
		Pro 5	1/8	7/7	5/22	3/—									—/2			2/6
		Val 6			7/14	—/1	—/11					1/6	3/2	—/1	9/11			5/2
		Glu 7				1/—												
		Lys 8																1/—
		Ser 9												4/3	1/3		1/—	15/17
		Ala 10												8/9				
		Thr 12																—/2
		Ala 13												1/1			1/3	—/1
		Leu 14												—/2				
		Lys 17														—/6		
	EF corner	Asp 79																
	GH corner	Glu 121													1/3			
	H helix	Pro 125									—/4							
		Val 126												1/3				

B. AXIAL CONTACTS

		1 or 2 α2						1 or 2 β2					
		A helix	B helix	G helix	GH corner			G helix		GH corner			
		Lys 16	His 20	His 112	Pro 114	Ala 115	Glu 116	His 116	His 117	Phe 118	Gly 119	Lys 120	Glu 121
α1 GH corner	Pro 114	—/7				—/1	7/6						
	Ala 115	—/5											
1 or 2 β1 A helix	Trp 15											1/1	
	Gly 16									2/—		12/7	1/2
	Lys 17			1/—	3/—			—/2	—/7	6/16	8/7	20/27	
	Val 18											4/16	
B helix	Asn 19			1/—								—/2	
	Glu 22		—/1										
G helix	His 116	—/10				1/—	1/—						
	His 117	—/3			23/8	4/1	—/1						
GH corner	Phe 118				31/13	10/3							
	Gly 119					5/—							
	Lys 120					—/2							
	Glu 121				4/5			—/3	—/4				

C. CONTACTS BETWEEN ANTIPARALLEL STRANDS

		2α1												
		CD corner		E helix			EF corner				F helix			
		His 45	Asp 47	Ala 53	Gln 54	Asn 68	His 72	Asp 75	Asn 78	Ala 79	Leu 80	Ser 81	Ala 82	Heme
1α1 CD corner	His 45					6	6			1				
	Phe 46						3							
	Asp 47												5	
E helix	Ala 53							7				1		
	Gln 54					1		22	19		1	1		
	Lys 61						11							
	Asn 68	6												
EF corner	His 72	4			3									1
	Asp 75			2										
	Asn 78			16	11									
	Ala 79				11									
F helix	Ala 82		1											
	Heme						10							

INDEX

169

---

*A complete list of abnormal hemoglobins (due to point mutations) is given in Table 4.3, pages 151–157, based on mutant data from the International Hemoglobin Information Center, Medical College of Georgia, Augusta, Georgia 30912. Updated lists of hemoglobin variants are issued periodically by this institution.